Amebiasis

Discard

Tropical Medicine: Science and Practice

Series Editors: Geoffrey Pasvol
Dept. of Infection & Tropical Medicine
Imperial College School of Medicine, UK

Stephen L Hoffman
Naval Medical Research Institute
Rockville, Maryland, USA

Published

Vol. 1   Lymphatic Filariasis
Edited by Thomas B Nutman

Forthcoming

Schistosomiasis
Edited by A Mahmoud

TROPICAL MEDICINE
Science and Practice
Volume 2

Amebiasis

edited by

Jonathan I Ravdin

Nesbitt Professor and Chairman
Department of Medicine
University of Minnesota Medical School

Series editors:
G Pasvol and SL Hoffman

Imperial College Press

ICP

Published by

Imperial College Press
57 Shelton Street
Covent Garden
London WC2H 9HE

Distributed by

World Scientific Publishing Co. Pte. Ltd.
P O Box 128, Farrer Road, Singapore 912805
USA office: Suite 1B, 1060 Main Street, River Edge, NJ 07661
UK office: 57 Shelton Street, Covent Garden, London WC2H 9HE

British Library Cataloguing-in-Publication Data
A catalogue record for this book is available from the British Library.

AMEBIASIS
Series on Tropical Medicine: Science and Practice — Vol. 2

Copyright © 2000 by Imperial College Press

ISBN   1-86094-133-8

This book is printed on acid-free paper.

Printed in Singapore by Regal Press (S) Pte. Ltd.

List of Contributors

A Bhattacharya
School of Life Sciences, Jawaharlal Nehru University
New Mehrauli Road, New Delhi 110 067, India
E-mail: alok@jnuniv.ernet.in

D Campbell
Department of Parasitology of McGill University
Macdonald Campus, 21,111 Lakeshore Rd.
Ste. Anne de Bellevue, Quebec, H9X 3V9, Canada

M Espinosa Cantellano
Departamento de Patología Experimental, CINVESTAV
Aptdo. Postal 14-740, CP 07000 México D.F., México
E-mail: mespinosa@pat.cinvestav.mx

K Chadee
Department of Parasitology of McGill University
Macdonald Campus, 21,111 Lakeshore Rd.
Ste. Anne de Bellevue, Quebec, H9X 3V9, Canada
E-mail: kris_chadee@maclan.mcgill.ca

CG Clark
Department of Infectious and Tropical Diseases
London School of Hygiene and Tropical Medicine
Keppel Street, London WC1E 7HT, UK
E-mail: graham.clark@lshtm.ac.uk

Terry FHG Jackson
South African Medical Research Council
P. O. Box 17120, Congella 4013, South Africa
E-mail: jacksont@mrc.ac.za

KC Kain
Tropical Disease Unit, EN G-224
Toronto General Hospital, 200 Elizabeth Street
Toronto, ON, Canada, M5G 2C4
E-mail: kkain@torhosp.toronto.on.ca

JS Keystone
Tropical Disease Unit, EN G-224
Toronto General Hospital, 200 Elizabeth Street
Toronto, ON, Canada, M5G 2C4

David Mirelman
The Besen-Brender Chair of Microbiology and Parasitology
Department of Biological Chemistry
The Weizmann Institute of Science
Rehovot 76100, Israel

WA Petri, Jr
Room 2115 MR4 Building, Lane Road
University of Virginia HSC, Charlottesville, VA 22908, USA
E-mail: wap3g@virginia.edu

DR Pillai
Tropical Disease Unit, EN G-224
Toronto General Hospital, 200 Elizabeth Street
Toronto, ON, Canada, M5G 2C4

G Ramakrishan
Room 2115 MR4 Building, Lane Road
University of Virginia HSC, Charlottesville, VA 22908, USA
E-mail: gr6q@virginia.edu

Jonathan I Ravdin, MD
Nesbitt Professor and Chairman
Department of Medicine, University of Minnesota Medical School
420 Delaware Street, S.E., Minneapolis, MN 55455, USA
E-mail: ravdin001@gold.tc.umn.edu

SL Reed
Departments of Pathology and Medicine
UCSD Medical Center, 200 W. Arbor Dr.
San Diego, Ca 92103-8416, USA
E-mail: slreed@ucsd.edu

SL Stanley, Jr
Department of Medicine and Molecular Microbiology
Washington, University School of Medicine
660 S. Euclid Avenue, St. Louis
MO, 63110 USA
E-mail: sstanley@im.wustl.edu

Contents

Chapter 1

Entamoeba Histolytica: An Overview of the Biology of the Organism

CG Clark

Department of Infectious and Tropical Diseases
London School of Hygiene and Tropical Medicine
Keppel Street, London WC1E 7HT, UK
E-mail: graham.clark@lshtm.ac.uk

M Espinosa Cantellano

Departamento de Patología Experimental, CINVESTAV
Aptdo. Postal 14-740, CP 07000 México D.F., México
E-mail: mespinosa@pat.cinvestav.mx

A Bhattacharya

School of Life Sciences, Jawaharlal Nehru University
New Mehrauli Road, New Delhi 110 067, India
E-mail: alok@jnuniv.ernet.in

Study of the biology of *Entamoeba histolytica* has a long history but the organism has not yet yielded all of its secrets. However, in the past several years significant advances have been made in our understanding of the parasite. This chapter briefly summarises our knowledge of the basic biology of *E. histolytica*, concentrating on the more recent discoveries.

Introduction

Organisms belonging to four genera of amoebae are recognised as colonising the human large intestine but *Entamoeba histolytica* is the only species unequivocally known to cause disease in humans. For this reason it is by far the most widely studied intestinal protistan parasite, with a literature spanning over 120 years. Comprehensive coverage of the basic biology of *E. histolytica* would require a book unto itself. Therefore this chapter will give an outline of the current status of the field and will concentrate on the most recent findings. Where appropriate, reference will be made to more complete reviews on specific areas of interest.

Taxonomy And Phylogeny

Entamoeba Taxonomy

The Early Years

The taxonomy of *E. histolytica* has a tortured history. The organism was first identified by Fedor Lösch working in St. Petersburg, Russia, in 1875 (1). He called it 'Amoeba coli' but did not give a formal taxonomic description. That honour fell to Fritz Schaudinn in 1903 (2) who created the species name *Entamoeba histolytica* for Lösch's amoeba but whose description of the life cycle contained many inaccuracies. Numerous additional parasitic amoeba species were described from humans in the following 15 years and it was not until the classic work by Clifford Dobell in 1919 (3) that the picture became clearer. Dobell recognised only three species of *Entamoeba* as being human parasites — *E. histolytica*, *E. coli* and *E. gingivalis*. All human infections involving an *Entamoeba* species producing cysts with four nuclei were ascribed to *E. histolytica*, those producing cysts with eight nuclei to *E. coli*, and all oral infections to *E. gingivalis*. All the other described human species of *Entamoeba* (and a few placed in other genera) were deemed to be synonyms of one of these three. This was the prevalent view for many years.

Entamoeba hartmanni

In 1912, von Prowazek (4) had described an organism he named *Entamoeba hartmanni*. This amoeba was morphologically similar to *E. histolytica* and also produced cysts with four nuclei but was smaller. Dobell (3) deemed it to be a synonym as the size range of *E. hartmanni* overlapped with that of *E. histolytica*. His view was widely accepted and remained so until the mid 1950's when Burrows (5) demonstrated that there were indeed minor but consistent morphological differences between the two and that, although the ranges overlapped, there were two distinct mean sizes. The existence of two forms had been recognised in the interim through reference to 'small race *E. histolytica*' in numerous publications. Subsequently, antigenic differences between *E. hartmanni* and *E. histolytica* were identified (6) and recently phylogenetic analysis has shown that the two are not very closely related (7, 8).

Entamoeba dispar

A second synonym took much longer to establish itself as a distinct entity. In 1925, Emile Brumpt (9) proposed that there were in fact two species within what was being called *E. histolytica*. One of these caused disease in humans and the other did not. The latter he named *Entamoeba dispar* and based his description solely on the relative ability of the two species to cause disease in humans and experimental animals. Because there was compelling evidence that *E. histolytica* isolated from some asymptomatic humans was capable of causing disease in other experimental subjects (10), and because the two species were morphologically indistinguishable, Brumpt's hypothesis was largely ignored for 50 years.[a]

In the interim, essentially only Brumpt and his student Tschedomir Simic used the species name *E. dispar*. Simic published several studies on the experimental infection of humans (11) and other mammals (12) with what he was calling *E. dispar* — no invasive disease was ever observed.

After Brumpt's death in 1951 the species name disappeared from the literature. However, in 1973 it was reported that amoebae isolated from patients with disease showed different lectin agglutination characteristics to those isolated from individuals with asymptomatic infections (13), the first biochemical evidence for subgroups within *E. histolytica*. Then, in 1978, it was reported that isoenzymes could distinguish two groups within *E. histolytica* that correlated with the disease status of the individual from whom the amoebae were isolated (14). Sargeaunt, Williams and colleagues went on to obtain data on thousands of *E. histolytica* isolates collected world-wide and showed that amoebae isolated from individuals with asymptomatic infections were almost always assigned to what they termed 'non-pathogenic zymodemes'. In contrast, those amoebae isolated from individuals with

[a]The fascinating discussion recorded following Brumpt's presentation to the Royal Society of Hygiene and Tropical Medicine in 1928 (279) sets forth most of the arguments that resulted in Brumpt's work being ignored for so long.

amoebic dysentery or amoebic liver abscess invariably gave the distinct isoenzyme patterns characteristic of 'pathogenic zymodemes' (15). As would be expected, a few asymptomatic carriers of 'pathogenic *E. histolytica*' were also identified. As early as 1982, Sargeaunt *et al.* (16) were already suggesting the possibility of the 'non-pathogenic *E. histolytica*' being synonymous with Brumpt's *E. dispar*.

Over the next 15 years evidence for the existence of two groups continued to accumulate and came to include antigenic differences (17) and genetic markers (18) in addition to isoenzymes. In 1993, *Entamoeba histolytica* was formally redescribed (19) to separate it from *E. dispar*, finally validating Brumpt's hypothesis after almost seventy years. This nomenclature now has been universally adopted in the field of amoebiasis research (20).

This change in nomenclature did not come about without controversy. In 1986, it was reported that the characteristic isoenzyme patterns of the two groups were not stable but were interconvertible (21, 22). This observation was later also made by others (23–26). Although subsequently shown to be an artefact (27), the 'conversion' observation has appeared in several textbooks where it is presented without qualification.

Entamoeba moshkovskii

Although never truly considered a synonym, *Entamoeba moshkovskii* is also morphologically indistinguishable from *E. histolytica*. Initially described from sewage in Russia (28), this species has subsequently been found to be common in anaerobic sediments world-wide, in fresh and brackish water, both clean and waste-contaminated.[b] It has remarkable osmotolerance and grows at a wide range of temperatures (29). It is also genetically diverse, with at least six distinct genetic lineages having been described (7). Its significance lies in occasional reports of human infections. These are very rare — about eight are known — but in one case, at least, the identity of the amoeba was not recognised initially and extensive experimental human infection and chemotherapy trials were undertaken[c] (30, 31). For many years known as '*E. histolytica*-like' amoebae, the true identity of these human isolates as *E. moshkovskii* was eventually established using DNA markers (32). It is interesting to note that only one of the six genetic lineages has ever been reported from human infections.

---

[b]Reviewed by Clark and Diamond (7, 32).
[c]The isolate is that known as 'Huff'.

Other Human Entamoeba Species

The other *Entamoeba* species known to infect humans are *E. coli*, which is probably the most common *Entamoeba* infection, *E. gingivalis*, the oral parasite, *E. polecki* and *E. chattoni*. The latter two species produce cysts with a single nucleus and are quite closely related[d] (8). Human infection with *E. chattoni* has only been reported in zookeepers (33) as its normal hosts are non-human primates. Pigs are the usual host for *E. polecki* and some link to these animals is commonly found when infected humans are identified (34). The lack of a cyst stage in *E. gingivalis* implies that direct transmission must be taking place, presumably through saliva. Occasional *E. gingivalis* infections of the uterus have been described but only in the presence of an intrauterine device and a bacterial infection (35). Genetic variants of both *E. gingivalis* and *E. coli* have been described (7), but their importance is purely academic. No disease in mammals has ever been reliably linked to *Entamoeba* species other than *E. histolytica*, although recently post-mortem invasion of tissue by *E. chattoni* was reported (36).

The Genus Entamoeba

In addition to the species nomenclature problems, the genus *Entamoeba* itself underwent a period of uncertainty. Beginning in 1928 a number of workers, primarily in North America, started using the genus name *Endamoeba* for these organisms in response to an opinion given by the International Commission on Zoological Nomenclature. Despite a stinging refutation of the Commission's arguments by Dobell (37) it was not until 1954 that the decision was reversed. The type species of the genus *Entamoeba* is *E. coli* having been described in 1895 by Casagrandi and Barbagallo.

Entamoeba Phylogeny

All species in the genus *Entamoeba* are characterised by a distinctive nuclear structure, among other characteristics, and so it came as no surprise when phylogenetic analysis of ribosomal RNA gene sequences confirmed the monophyletic nature of the genus (8). In addition, the three groups of species classically identified by the number of nuclei in their mature cyst

---

[d]Some authorities have considered them to be synonyms.

proved to be monophyletic (7, 8). Within the group of species that produces cysts with four nuclei, the three morphologically indistinguishable species *E. histolytica*, *E. dispar* and *E. moshkovskii* also proved to be genetically the most similar to each other, with *E. histolytica* and *E. dispar* being sibling species (7). The degree of genetic divergence between *E. histolytica* and *E. dispar* is not insignificant, however, approximating that between humans and mice. The three species in which intraspecific genetic variation has been found — *E. coli*, *E. gingivalis* and *E. moshkovskii* — illustrate some of the problems associated with the species concept in organisms that are primarily, if not exclusively, asexual. The degree of genetic divergence among variants of both *E. coli* and *E. moshkovskii* exceeds that between *E. histolytica* and *E. dispar*.

The lineage leading to *Entamoeba* has no clearly identifiable relatives among free-living protists but in most analyses the parasitic amoeba *Endolimax nana* appears to be distantly related (8). In contrast to the expectations of some researchers (38, 39), there is no evidence for *Entamoeba* being a 'primitive' eukaryote. The implication from ribosomal DNA and certain other gene sequence analyses is that the genus diverged from other eukaryotes later than some organisms with more 'typical' eukaryotic cell structure (see below). This finding means that many of the unusual characteristics of *Entamoeba* species must have arisen through secondary loss, perhaps in response to parasitism, rather than having been primitively absent.

Formal Description of Entamoeba histolytica

The following description of *E. histolytica*, mostly at the light microscope level, closely mirrors that of Diamond and Clark (19) but none of the essential features recorded has changed since the description of Dobell in 1919 (3) with the exception of the size ranges (due to the exclusion of *E. hartmanni*). It is also based on organisms isolated directly from the host; *E. histolytica* in axenic culture has a quite different appearance.

Trophozoite

This ranges in size from 20 μm to 40 μm in diameter. Locomotion is by means of a single well defined pseudopodium, often extended eruptively, without clear differentiation between ectoplasm and endoplasm. There is normally a single nucleus. The cytoplasm often has ingested red blood cells when the trophozoites are isolated from symptomatic individuals. Sometimes leukocytes and bacteria are visible. The cytoplasm is rich in glycogen and has ribosomes arranged in helices which aggregate. There are no classical mitochondria, rough endoplasmic reticulum, or Golgi apparatus visible. The nucleus is spherical, measuring 4 μm to 7 μm in diameter, consisting of a delicate achromatic membrane lined usually by a single layer of small chromatin granules, uniform in size, in contact or very close to each other. The nucleus has a small spherical karyosome (0.5 μm in diameter), often centrally located, surrounded by an achromatic capsule-like structure.

Cysts

These are spherical, measuring 10 μm to 16 μm in diameter, with four nuclei when mature. Glycogen is present in a distinct vacuole in the immature cyst, but this becomes more diffuse as the cyst matures. Immature cysts often contain chromatoid bodies made of ribosomes that aggregate to form characteristically shaped elongate bars with rounded ends. These disappear as the cyst matures. Cyst nuclei are morphologically similar to those of trophozoites, but are smaller in the mature cyst.

Geographic Distribution

World-wide.

Hosts

Humans appear to be the primary host, but several non-human primates, cats, dogs and rats have also been documented as occasional hosts. Reports of infection in other mammals must be viewed with caution if based on morphology alone.

Differentiation of E. histolytica from E. dispar

There are no consistent morphological differences between E. *histolytica* and E. *dispar*. The initial in vitro method for differentiation of E. *histolytica* from E. *dispar* was based on a single isoenzyme pattern (phosphoglucomutase) (14) but the number of enzymes that give a species specific pattern has now grown to seven (40) and the most widely used enzyme is hexokinase. Numerous antigenic differences have now been described and the sequences of almost every gene studied to date have proven to be distinct.[e] Isoenzyme patterns remain the 'gold standard' for distinguishing the two species but more rapid and sensitive methods based on antigen detection and DNA amplification have now been described.[f] In addition to the above mentioned differences, the relative ability of *E. histolytica* and *E. dispar* to grow under axenic conditions (41) is a very distinctive feature (see below).

The described differences between *E. histolytica* and *E. dispar* do not easily explain why one causes disease in humans and the other does not. There are two cysteine protease genes (42) and one antigen gene family (43) that are present only in *E. histolytica* but for the most part the differences between the two species are quantitative rather than qualitative. One explanation suggested for why *E. histolytica* causes disease is that it is a relatively recent member of the human parasite fauna and is not yet fully adapted to this host (44).

Cultivation

Cultivation with bacteria

Entamoeba histolytica was first cultivated in vitro by Boeck and Drbohlav in 1925 (45), to the surprise of Dobell who had viewed it up to that time as being an obligate tissue parasite (3). The cultivation was accidental, as the experiment had been set up to isolate intestinal flagellates. The medium was diphasic, a slant of inspissated egg overlaid with a saline solution and serum. This medium, with minor modifications, is still in use today. Numerous other media for the cultivation of *E. histolytica* in the presence of a mixed bacterial flora (xenic cultures) have been described (reviewed by Diamond (46)), but the most widely used are the diphasic Robinson's medium (47) and the monophasic TYSGM-9 (48).

---

[e]The differences described up to 1993 are summarised in the redescription paper (19) but many more have been, and continue to be, reported.
[f]A large number of such reports have been published. Among the more recent are these (280–284).

Axenic cultivation

Attempts to grow *E. histolytica* in the absence of any other organisms (axenically) were made by many prominent parasitologists but it was not until the work of Louis Diamond in 1961 (49) that this was finally achieved. It is not clear in retrospect why he was successful when others had failed but his approach has been the method employed for axenisation of *Entamoeba* isolates ever since. The xenic *E. histolytica* is grown first in monoxenic culture with a kinetoplastid flagellate and antibiotics (50) followed by a gradual weaning of the amoebae from this food source. The original axenic culture medium he developed (49) was diphasic and it was complex to make and use. In 1968 the first monophasic medium for axenic cultivation of *E. histolytica* (TPS-1) was described by Diamond (51) and this was accompanied by a significantly improved yield of cells and ease of handling which together dramatically opened up the possibilities in certain areas of research. TPS-1 was superseded in 1978 by TYI-S-33 (52). Other media for axenic culture have been described but TYI-S-33 is by far the most widely used today.

One observation regarding *E. dispar* is appropriate at this point. While *E. dispar* grows just as well as *E. histolytica* in xenic cultures, the same is not true of monoxenic or axenic cultivation. Monoxenic cultures of *E. dispar* can be obtained but their growth is usually much inferior to *E. histolytica* under identical conditions. Likewise, axenic cultivation of *E. dispar* proved very difficult and there have still only been two reported successes (41, 53), which required use of different media (53, 54). This profound difference in axenic growth potential is one of the characteristics that separates the two species. It has been proposed that these growth differences are in part due to the relative ability of the two organisms to obtain nutrients by pinocytosis rather than by phagocytosis (the method used in xenic culture and in the host) (41). This has been supported by recent scanning electron microscope studies which show that axenic *E. dispar* trophozoites have very few pinocytotic vesicle openings in the plasma membrane (see below).

Biochemistry

With a few notable exceptions, basic biochemistry studies in *E. histolytica* have been rather scant in the last 15 to 20 years. The review by Reeves (55) remains the single best source for biochemical information on this organism. More recently, insights into basic biochemistry often have been the result of genetic studies. Three independent Expressed Sequence Tag (EST) analyses of *E. histolytica* (56–58) and one study of *E. dispar* ESTs (59) have recently added greatly to our knowledge. EST analyses involve partial sequencing of randomly chosen clones from a cDNA library followed by comparison of the sequence obtained with those already deposited in sequence databases. Many of the EST gene identifications must still be considered tentative as they are often based solely on similarity of the deduced sequence to previously identified heterologous genes in the database. Where more appropriate, information from the EST studies has been integrated into other sections of this chapter.

Intermediary Metabolism

In vitro, *E. histolytica* is essentially an aerotolerant anaerobe. It respires and consumes a small amount of oxygen. However, it may be sensitive to the higher level of oxygen and reactive oxygen species it encounters when it invades tissues. Two known *E. histolytica* enzymes can generate hydrogen peroxide: the NADPH-flavin oxidoreductase (60, 61) and the iron containing superoxide dismutase (62, 63). Catalase is not present (55) and neither is glutathione or trypanothione (64, 65). Hydrogen peroxide is thought to be degraded by a thiol-dependent peroxidase (66, 67), previously known as the 29 kDa/30 kDa cysteine-rich antigen. The presence of a gene encoding cystathionine-γ-synthase in *E. dispar* (59) indicates that the thiol containing metabolite cystathionine may be present and may help in detoxification of oxygen and reactive oxygen species. Cystathionine-γ-synthase is also the first enzyme in the biosynthesis of amino acid methionine. There is also evidence to suggest that cysteine is synthesised in *E. histolytica* as genes encoding cysteine synthase (68), serine acetyltransferase and ATP-sulfurylase (69) have been identified. Cysteine synthase is cytoplasmic and exists in two isoforms (68). However, cysteine appears to be an essential amino acid for growth of *E. histolytica* (70). The presence of significantly higher intracellular levels of glutamate and proline than in the growth medium may indicate the ability to synthesise these amino acids also (71). So far there is no information about metabolic pathways involving other amino acids, other than a list of essential and non-essential amino acids determined empirically during development of the partially defined medium PDM-805 (70).

Carbohydrates are the main energy source for the parasite. The pathway involved in the fermentation of glucose includes some unusual enzymes that use pyrophosphate (PPi) rather than a nucleoside triphosphate as the phosphate donor (55). Many of the genes encoding enzymes of the glycolytic pathway have been cloned and sequenced. Phylogenetic analysis of some of these suggests that they may be of bacterial origin and thus may have been acquired by horizontal transfer (72). This conclusion requires further confirmation as the number of gene sequences available from distinct species for some enzymes is quite small.

Both D-glucose and D-galactose are transported and actively metabolised by *E. histolytica* (55). A cDNA encoding the enzyme galactokinase, the first enzyme in the galactose utilisation pathway, has been detected in glucose-grown *E. histolytica* (56) suggesting that this enzyme may be expressed constitutively, consistent with earlier biochemical observations (55). Galactose enters the glycolytic pathway via glycogen which is present at high levels in axenic *E. histolytica* (30 mM glucose equivalents (71)). Identification of genes encoding glycogen phosphorylase (57) and phosphoglucomutase (73) and the detection of the necessary uridyl transferase and epimerase activities (55) suggest that *E. histolytica* and *E. dispar* may have a pathway for glycogen metabolism similar to that of the mammalian system. The presence of both α- and β- amylase activities (74) and the unusually compact structure of *E. histolytica* glycogen (71) have been documented.

In the glycolytic pathway, genes encoding glucokinase (hexokinase) (75), two phosphofructokinases (PPi dependent) (76-78), triosephosphate isomerase (79), glyceraldehyde-3-phosphate dehydrogenase (56, 57), enolase (80, 81), pyruvate phosphate dikinase (82, 83), phosphoglyceromutase (58), ferredoxin (84) and pyruvate:ferredoxin oxidoreductase (85, 86) have been identified. From acetyl-CoA, ethanol is produced by action of acetate thiokinase (87), a bifunctional acetaldehyde/alcohol dehydrogenase (88, 89) and a NADP dependent alcohol dehydrogenase (90–92). All these enzymes have been reported to be non-sedimentable, implying a cytoplasmic location (55). One report of a membrane bound pyruvate:ferredoxin oxidoreductase needs to be replicated (93).

Oxygen consumption is stimulated by glucose (94) but this pathway is almost completely unknown. The presence of ubiquinone in *E. histolytica* has been demonstrated (95) and this may well accept electrons from ferredoxin, but the subsequent pathway to oxygen, if indeed oxygen is the terminal acceptor, is unknown. While the terminal acceptor may be oxygen when oxygen is present, the terminal acceptor under anaerobic conditions is completely unknown. Given that *E. histolytica* has no detectable haem iron (96), cytochromes are not involved. The relative levels of NAD^+, $NADP^+$,

NADH, NADPH and ATP molecules are likely to be very important in *E. histolytica* due to the lack of a mitochondrial electron transport chain and tricarboxylic acid cycle. The gene encoding adenylate kinase has been reported (56, 57). Adenylate kinase maintains ATP balance within the cell by interconversion of AMP, ATP and ADP. It can generate energy not only from the high energy γ-phosphate but also the β-phosphate which may be significant for this organism. The balance among the different forms of pyridine nucleotides may be maintained in part by the enzyme pyridine nucleotide transhydrogenase (97–99) which catalyses hydrogen exchange between the two nucleotides (NAD and NADP).

Little is known of nucleic acid metabolism in *E. histolytica*. It is a purine auxotroph but can apparently synthesise pyrimidines (55). Likewise little is known about lipid metabolism. At least three phospholipase activities (A1, A2 and L1) have been detected (100, 101). *E. histolytica* appears able to synthesise at least some of its lipids (for example ceramide aminoethyl phosphonate, which is presumably absent from the medium) but details are scarce. Recent results indicate an ability to synthesise cholesterol (in contrast to earlier reports) and isoprenoids (102). The only detectable polyamine present is putrescine, at 9.5 mM (71). As it is present in only trace amounts in the growth medium it must therefore be synthesised by the amoeba, and perhaps acts as an osmolyte (71). Enzymes involved in inositol metabolism have been identified (103, 104), as have some of the early enzymes in the biosynthesis of glycosylated proteins (105, 106).

Protein Turnover

Cysteine proteases are the most abundant proteases present in *E. histolytica* and have also been implicated in its virulence (107). Four major cysteine proteases of 56 kDa (108), 26–29 kDa (109, 110), 22–27 kDa (111) and a 16 kDa cathepsin B-like (112) have been reported. The relationships among these molecules have not been completely worked out. Genes encoding six distinct cysteine proteases have been cloned from *E. histolytica* and four have been detected in *E. dispar* (42). Genes encoding cysteine proteases have also been characterised from *E. invadens* (113). Among other proteases, a gene encoding a homologue of the calcium regulated protease calpain (57) and a proteosome complex (114) have also been identified. The proteosome is an intracellular complex of proteins involved in the degradation of ubiquitin-conjugated intracellular proteins with a variety of cellular functions. Genes encoding ubiquitin (115) and four different proteosome subunits, α- (116), S2- (117), ι- and DD5 (in *E. dispar* (59)) have been identified and a ubiquitin conjugating system (118) is also known to exist, showing that this intracellular pathway for protein degradation is present in *Entamoeba*. The intracellular amino acid pools of *E. histolytica* have been studied using NMR spectroscopy (71). While the levels of most amino acids are similar to those in the culture medium, some are present at higher concentrations intracellularly than in the medium, indicating either preferential concentration or synthesis of these amino acids.

Cell Biology

The life cycle

With few exceptions, all *Entamoeba* species have a simple life cycle consisting of an infective cyst stage and a multiplying trophozoite stage. Within the genus *Entamoeba*, species variously produce cysts with one, four or eight nuclei. There is no cyst stage in a few species, for example *E. gingivalis*, but this appears to be the result of secondary loss of this feature (8).

In *E. histolytica* the mature cyst contains four nuclei. The cyst is ingested in faecally contaminated food or water and passes through the stomach and small intestine.[g] The trophozoite emerges in the terminal ileum or as the cyst enters the large intestine[h] where it establishes the new infection. The process of excystation has been studied both in vitro (119) and in monkeys (120) with essentially identical results. The first stage involves movement of the amoeba within the cyst wall. This is followed by a thinning of the wall at one point through which the amoeba emerges, usually after numerous extensions and retractions of pseudopodia, leaving behind an empty cyst wall. The multi-nucleated trophozoite may start feeding even before fully emerging from the cyst. The four-nucleated amoeba[i] undergoes three rounds of cytokinesis and one round of nuclear division to give rise to eight daughter amoebae (119). Trophozoites ingest bacteria and multiply by binary fission

---

[g]Since cultures can be established from cysts *in vitro* without simulating passage through the stomach (i.e. without treatment with hydrochloric acid) this must not be an obligate signal to initiate excystation. It is not clear what the signal is but it could involve the action of host enzymes on the cyst wall.

[h]This is by extrapolation to humans from data obtained in non-human primates (120).

[i]Immature cysts can also excyst (120) although it is not known whether they can establish new infections.

in the colon where, in response to unknown stimuli, they re-encyst.[j] Cysts are shed periodically in the stool thus completing the cycle.

Trophozoites are short-lived outside the body and do not survive passage through the upper gastrointestinal tract. In contrast, cysts may remain viable in a humid environment and stay infective for several days. The invasive form of the parasite is the trophozoite which can penetrate the intestinal mucosa and disseminate to other organs. Cysts do not develop within tissues. Strictly speaking tissue invasion is not part of the life cycle as those organisms that pass across the mucosa are no longer capable of giving rise to new infections. Invasive disease must therefore be viewed as aberrant behaviour on the part of the organism.

DNA synthesis during encystation and excystation has not been studied in *E. histolytica* but by extrapolation from the reptilian species *E. invadens* it is likely that there is only one round of DNA replication[k] (121). It does not appear that any DNA synthesis occurs during excystation.[l] Therefore, if there is only one round of DNA replication through encystment and excystment, the ploidy of the trophozoite before encystation must be at least $4n$ to give rise to eight $1n$ daughter amoebae. This is in agreement with a recent report indicating a functional ploidy of at least $4n$ in *E. histolytica* (122).

The cyst

Cysts have been studied far less than trophozoites, mainly due to our inability to induce encystation of *E. histolytica* in axenic cultures. Thus, many studies on *Entamoeba* cysts have been on *E. invadens*, a parasite of reptiles which can be made to encyst in culture (123). *E. histolytica* cysts are round or slightly oval hyaline bodies 10 μm–16 μm in diameter. They are surrounded by a refractile wall, 125–150 nm thick, which appears to be made of fibrillar material forming a tight mesh that may give rise to several lamellae. In *E. invadens* the cyst wall has been shown to contain chitin. Chitinases hydrolyse chitin polymers present in the cyst wall. Recently, the chitinase genes of *E. histolytica*, *E. dispar* and *E. invadens* have been cloned (124), but expression has been detected only in encysting *E. invadens*. The plasma

---

[j]Although encystation stimuli are unknown, galactose and N-acetyl glucosamine have been reported to inhibit encystation in *E. invadens* (285).
[k]This is supported by observed changes in nuclear volume.
[l]Again this is supported by the observed decrease in nuclear volume.

membrane frequently has deep invaginations; polyribosomes and vacuoles containing dense fibrogranular material can be observed close to its cytoplasmic face, while food vacuoles tend to disappear as the cyst matures. When stained with iron-hematoxylin, the cyst cytoplasm appears vacuolated with numerous glycogen deposits that decrease in size and number as the cyst matures. Chromatoid bodies, which are aggregated ribosomes, can be identified inside the cytoplasm as rod shaped structures with blunt or rounded ends. A number of cyst wall antigens have been identified using monoclonal antibodies but they have not yet been further characterised (125).

The trophozoite

The trophozoite of *E. histolytica* is a highly dynamic and pleomorphic cell, whose form and motility are greatly affected by changes in temperature, pH, osmolarity and redox potential. The axenisation of *E. dispar* trophozoites has allowed a detailed morphological and ultrastructural comparison with *E. histolytica* under identical conditions (126). Although there was no single feature present in all amoebae that could be used to distinguish one species from another, subtle differences between the two parasites were observed and will be mentioned below. Unless *E. dispar* is specifically mentioned, the description applies to both species. It should be remembered that organisms isolated from the host or grown in xenic culture may not share all of the characteristics described below.

The overall shape of *E. dispar* is elongated, with a prominent, broad, anterior pseudopod, and a distinct, posterior uroid that appears as a tail formed of irregular folds of the membrane and thread-like processes called filopodia. In contrast, *E. histolytica* trophozoites in axenic culture tend to be rounder in shape, have several small pseudopodia extending from different parts of the cell, and a uroid is less commonly observed (126). Filopodia can also be found in other regions of the cell surface and are more frequently observed on amoebae in monoxenic cultures or in contact with epithelial tissues (127).

The diameter of the cell varies between 10 μm–60 μm not only due to the pleomorphism of the parasite, but also dependent on the feeding conditions: amoebae obtained directly from intestinal or liver lesions are generally larger (20 μm–40 μm) than those found in nondysenteric stools or in cultures (10 μm–30 μm). When observed by scanning electron microscopy, the cell surface of *E. histolytica* appears rough, with numerous

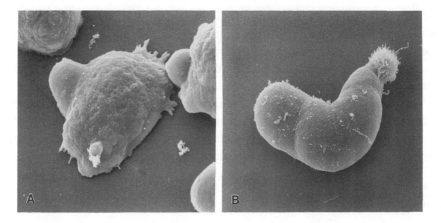

Figure 1. Scanning electron micrographs of E. *histolytica* and E. *dispar* in axenic culture. The pleomorphic shape with several pseudopodia and a rough cell surface characteristic of E. *histolytica* trophozoites (A) is compared to the elongated form with a single pseudopodium, distinct uroid and smooth cell surface characteristic of most E. *dispar* trophozoites (B). Magnification X 2,000 (Courtesy of Dr. Bibiana Chávez).

circular openings 0.2 μm–0.4 μm in diameter that correspond to the mouths of micropinocytic vesicles. These openings are absent from the large protruding stomata of macropinocytic channels (2 μm–6 μm in diameter) and from pseudopodia. In contrast, the cell surface of E. *dispar* trophozoites has a smoother appearance (Figure 1) (126).

The nucleus

The nucleus of E. *histolytica* is 4 μm–7 μm in diameter. The nuclear membrane appears as a double membrane, interrupted by numerous nuclear pores approximately 65 nm in diameter. In E. *dispar* the thin peripheral rim of the nucleus is made up of regularly deposited dense granules of circular profile, whereas in E. *histolytica* the nuclear periphery is coarse and thick. Chromatin clumps are usually uniform in size and evenly distributed inside the nuclear membrane although in some cells the chromatin appears concentrated on one side as a crescent-shaped mass. The karyosome or endosome is a small spherical mass approximately 0.5 μm in diameter, located in the central part of the nucleus. In situ hybridisation experiments have identified the ribosomal RNA genes of *E. histolytica* in the peripheral chromatin (128). The karyosome is therefore not equivalent to the nucleolus of other eukaryotes. Intranuclear bodies 0.2 μm–1.0 μm in diameter are frequently observed but their nature and function are unknown.

Genes encoding histones are present in *E. histolytica* — H1, H2A, H2B, H3 and H4 have all been identified (57, 58, 129–131). Histones H3 and H2B have also been identified in *E. dispar* (59, 131). In *E. invadens* a polyadenylated form of histone H2B mRNA has been observed and expression of this mRNA is developmentally regulated (132). The chromatin structure of *E. histolytica* is not clear although some form of nucleosomal structure is thought to be present (133). *E. histolytica* chromatin does not condense and this may be due either to the divergent nature of the histones (129, 130) or to some property of the non-histone chromatin proteins.[m] More information is needed before any definite conclusions can be made.

Nuclear division proceeds without dissolution of the nuclear membrane and involves the participation of a thick microtubule spindle. Individual microtubules can be identified in cryofixed and cryosubstituted samples (134). In eukaryotic cells microtubules are organised around one or more microtubule organising centres (MTOC) or centrosomes which have gamma tubulins along with other proteins. A gene encoding γ-tubulin, a protein specifically associated with MTOCs, has been identified (135). An antibody against this γ-tubulin identified multiple perinuclear bodies, likely to be MTOCs, in trophozoites but these were not limited to dividing parasites. There is a need for further work in defining the role of these multiple MTOCs in nuclear division. With DNA-binding fluorescent dyes, six DNA-containing plaques can be seen in dividing nuclei, possibly corresponding to some of the organism's chromosomes (136, 137).

The doubling time during exponential growth in axenic culture has been calculated for one isolate of *E. histolytica* to be 8.7 hours (138), but little is known about the molecular mechanisms controlling growth and proliferation of the parasite (139). Several homologues of genes involved in regulation of the cell division cycle and signal transduction pathways in other eukaryotic cells have been isolated from *E. histolytica*: Eh *cdc2* (140), Eh *ras*, Eh *rap* (141), Eh *mfk*1 (142), and Eh *rho* (143). However, their role in *E. histolytica* has yet to be confirmed.

---

[m] The existence of non-histone chromatin proteins has yet to be demonstrated in *E. histolytica*.

The cytoplasm

In general, eukaryotic cells have numerous, functionally distinct, membrane-bound organelles that can be distinguished to some extent at the ultrastructural level. The functional identities of these organelles are defined by the presence of unique sets of enzymes and other proteins. The cytoplasm of *E. histolytica* trophozoites is notable for the apparent absence in transmission electron microscopy of most of the typical organelles found in other eukaryotic cells, i.e. mitochondria, Golgi apparatus, rough endoplasmic reticulum, centrioles and microtubules. Instead, the cytoplasm contains abundant vacuoles that are extremely variable in size, ranging from 0.5 μm to 9.0 μm in diameter. Such studies cannot rule out the possibility that functionally similar but structurally distinct organelle-like compartments could be present in the cytoplasm of these cells. Indeed recent studies suggest that these do exist (see below).

Preliminary studies comparing *E. histolytica* and *E. dispar* have revealed differences in the distribution of the vacuoles in the cytoplasm of the two species, by light and electron microscopy. The cytoplasm of *E. dispar* appears patchy: vacuoles are concentrated in some regions, while other areas, devoid of vacuoles, stain differently with Toluidine blue. In contrast, vacuoles in *E. histolytica* are larger and have a uniform distribution throughout the cytoplasm. A prominent feature of most *E. dispar* trophozoites studied by transmission electron microscopy is the existence of cytoplasmic areas containing large deposits of glycogen granules interspersed with ribosomal bundles (126); the glycogen may be responsible for the altered staining mentioned above (Figure 2).

Some of the vacuoles have been identified ultrastructurally and/or biochemically and include phagocytic vacuoles, macro- and micropinocytic vacuoles, lysosomes, residual bodies and autophagic vacuoles. Food vacuoles can be observed, filled with starch or bacteria when in amoebae from xenic cultures and kinetoplastids when from monoxenic cultures, and when recovered from dysenteric stools they often contain ingested red blood cells. The lysosomes of amoebae differ from those of other eukaryotes in that the enzymes they contain are bound to the lysosomal membrane rather than being free in the vacuolar compartment (reviewed by Martínez-Palomo (144)). A gene encoding the enzyme β-N-acetyl hexosaminidase has been isolated from *E. histolytica* (145). This enzyme is normally located in the lysosomes of other eukaryotic cells but its location in *E. histolytica* is not known.

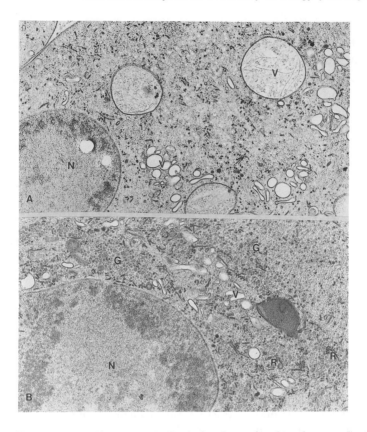

Figure 2. Transmission electron micrograph of cryofixed and cryosubstituted *E. histolytica* and *E. dispar* trophozoites.

In *E. histolytica* (A) a heterogeneous population of vacuoles uniformly distributed throughout the cytoplasm is seen. In *E. dispar* (B) the cytoplasmic vacuoles are generally smaller and concentrated in certain regions of the cytoplasm, while other areas are occupied by large deposits of glycogen granules interspersed with ribosome bundles. N = Nucleus; R = Ribosome bundles; G = Glycogen granules; V = Vacuoles. Magnification X 14,000 (Courtesy of Dr. Bibiana Chávez).

Our knowledge of this complex vacuolar system is mainly of the vacuoles involved in endocytic processes. The nature and functions of other vacuoles remain largely unknown and await further analysis. However, genes encoding proteins involved in vesicle formation in the trans-Golgi network, such as *E. dispar* clathrin heavy chain (59), *E. histolytica* clathrin coat assembly protein, dynamin and β-adaptin (56) are present. These proteins almost certainly participate in the formation of coated-pit-like structures observed in the plasma membrane of cryofixed and cryosubstituted trophozoites (Figure 3) (134). Small GTP-binding proteins of the *rab* family regulate specific vesicle targeting and/or fusion with the appropriate membrane targets. Five members of this family have been found in *E. histolytica* (*rab*7 (57), *rab*1a, *rab*8b (58), *rab*A and *rab*11 (146)) and may be specifically involved in trafficking from late endosomes to vacuoles.

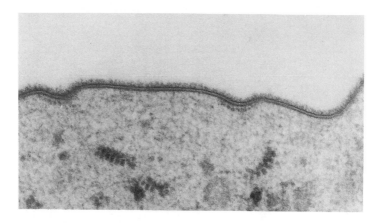

Figure 3. Transmission electron micrograph of an *E. histolytica* trophozoite. For the first time, coated-pit-like structures can be identified in the plasma membrane of cryofixed and cryosubstituted samples. Magnification X 149,000 (Courtesy of Dr. Arturo González-Robles).

The acidic pH of vacuoles is maintained by specific vacuolar-type H$^+$ ATPases, and such an enzyme has been characterised from *E. histolytica* (147–149). This enzyme, along with phosphoinositide 3-kinase and p21^{racA}, a *ras* family GTP-binding protein, was found to be involved in phagocytosis of bacteria and erythrocytes, consistent with a vacuolar function of these proteins (150). Cytoplasmic granules containing *E. histolytica* porins (amoebapores) and a novel class of lysozyme with two isoforms are thought to be released into these acidic vacuoles (151–153). *E. histolytica* has a high rate of endocytosis and recycling of plasma membrane components. Delivery of endocytic vesicles must be important for maintenance of vacuolar structure.

A lattice of tubules and vesicles superficially resembling smooth endoplasmic reticulum (ER) can very occasionally be found in the cytoplasm of *E. histolytica* trophozoites. The lattice is made up of extremely thin tubules of approximately 20 nm in diameter forming irregular whorls or parallel arrays. In contrast to the 10 nm thick plasma and vacuolar membranes, the membrane enclosing these tubules is only 6 nm thick (127). In other eukaryotes, protein movement from the cytosol to the ER involves the signal recognition particle (SRP). A gene encoding a protein constituent of this particle has been identified in *E. histolytica* (154) and amino-terminal signal peptides are known to be processed (155), indicating that even though an ultrastructural ER is difficult to identify a functional equivalent is indeed present. This is further supported by the presence of glycosylated and glycosylphosphatidylinositol anchored proteins in *E. histolytica* (156). The enzymes that perform these modifications are usually ER and/or Golgi resident. Ultrastructural evidence from cytochemical stains and fluorescent dyes also supports the existence of a Golgi-equivalent compartment (157, 158). A gene encoding a protein with characteristics of a protein disulphide isomerase has also been reported (159). Normally this protein is located in the ER. However, the *E. histolytica* protein does not have the typical tetrapeptide signal (KDEL) usually needed for retention in the ER, although this is also absent from the *Dictyostelium discoideum* protein (160). Occasionally, ER resident proteins may reach the cis-Golgi through vesicular traffic. ERD2 helps to retrieve these molecules from the cis-Golgi. The presence of this protein (161) suggests that *E. histolytica* may have vesicular traffic between ER and cis-Golgi comparable to that in other eukaryotes.

A recent report (162) used DNA transfection technology and heterologous antibodies to identify components of the secretory pathway in *E. histolytica*. The *E. histolytica* ER-resident chaperone BiP does have the KDEL ER retention signal and this was shown to be functional when attached to a protein that is normally secreted. Staining for this protein identified a small number of variably sized vesicles in the cytoplasm as being the ER equivalent, and targeting to this compartment is dependent on the presence of an amino-terminal signal peptide. Heterologous antibodies to mammalian Golgi-resident proteins identified a few, large, Brefeldin-A sensitive, perinuclear vesicles as being the Golgi equivalent in *E. histolytica*, similar to what is seen by cytochemistry (157, 158).

The *E. histolytica* genome encodes proteins that are normally associated with mitochondria in eukaryotes, yet nothing resembling a classical mitochondrion is seen in the amoeba cytoplasm. The molecular chaperones cpn60 (99) and mt-hsp70 (163) exhibit specific sequence similarity to mitochondrial homologues. Both the predicted chaperones and the pyridine nucleotide transhydrogenase (another protein normally associated with mitochondria in eukaryotes) genes appear to encode signal peptide-like sequences at the amino termini of the proteins (98, 99, 163, 164), and the transhydrogenase enzyme activity is sedimentable (97). Two recent reports have identified the compartment to which cpn60 is targeted in *E. histolytica* (variously called 'Crypton' (165) and 'mitosome' (166)). The organelles are oval, 1–2 μm in size and are usually present in only 1–2 copies per cell. Targeting of proteins to the compartment is dependent on short amino-terminal signal peptides that can be replaced with authentic mitochondrial targeting sequences (166). Although the current function of this organelle is unknown all the evidence points to it being of mitochondrial origin.

Cytoplasmic ribosomes appear to be found mostly in helical arrays approximately 300 nm in length and 40 nm in diameter. In cysts and resting cultured trophozoites the helices aggregate into large crystalline inclusions that can be several micrometers in length in the cyst, forming the classical chromatoid body with an hexagonal packing pattern. In the cyst these are clearly visible in the light microscope when stained with, for example, iron haematoxylin. (See below for ribosome-related genes)

The cytoskeleton

Despite the striking motility and plasticity of the trophozoite, little is known about the structural organisation of its cytoskeleton. Actin is the most abundant cytoskeletal protein. Under the transmission electron microscope, cryofixed and cryosubstituted trophozoites show microfilaments, 7 nm in diameter, located immediately below the plasma membrane and concentrated in pseudopodia and phagocytic stomata. Immunofluorescent staining with monoclonal antibodies and phalloidin have confirmed that these correspond to actin. At least four actin genes have been identified in the trophozoite, apparently encoding a single actin isoform of 45 kDa (167, 168). The most striking difference with many other reported actins is the inability of *Entamoeba* actin to interact with DNase I (169; this is also a characteristic of *Naegleria* actin (170)). The presence of accessory proteins that regulate the organisation of actin has only recently been investigated (171). The actin binding proteins identified include: myosin II and actin binding protein (ABP) 120, which seem to participate in cell locomotion in *E. histolytica* (172–174); myosin I, known to participate in the intracellular transport of vesicles, pinocytosis, phagocytosis and pseudopod extension (175–177); profilin, which has been described as regulating actin polymerisation and acting as a buffer to keep the effective concentration of free actin at a constant level $(178)^n$; vinculin, a component of adhesion plaques and desmosomes (175); α-actinin and tropomyosin, which have been identified in stress fibres in mammalian cells (175); F-actin capping protein, which binds to the end of actin filaments and prevents the addition or loss of actin monomers (58); and elongation factor (EF)-1α, which is capable of binding to and cross-linking actin and is an abundant protein in both *E. histolytica* and *E. dispar* (56-59). The possible function and assembly of these actin binding proteins during locomotion in *E. histolytica* will be discussed below.

Electron microscopic analysis of cryofixed and cryosubstituted trophozoites of *E. histolytica* has confirmed the absence of microtubules in both the cytoplasm and nuclei of non-dividing amoebae, and their presence only in the nuclei of dividing trophozoites (179). Microtubules are filaments of a heterodimer composed of α- and β-tubulin, polymerised by binding of the acidic C-terminal region of one tubulin dimer with the N-terminal region of another. Genes encoding α- and β-tubulin of *E. histolytica* have been isolated (180, 181). Although tubulins are in general very conserved proteins, the deduced amino acid sequences of these proteins in *E. histolytica* have proven highly divergent, with α-tubulin showing only 51–55% identity with the human, *Plasmodium* and *Saccharomyces* sequences, and β-tubulin having only 54–58% identity to the human, *Plasmodium*, *Trypanosoma*, *Leishmania*, and *Giardia* sequences (180, 181). Interestingly, the C-terminal region of *E. histolytica* α-tubulin is less acidic when compared to other α-tubulin sequences, which could affect the efficient polymerisation of tubulin dimers and explain the difficulty in visualising microtubules in *E. histolytica* (181).

The finding of cylindrical particles in the cytoplasm of *E. histolytica* has generated considerable interest. They are found in trophozoites obtained from such diverse sources as colonic exudates from individuals with acute amoebic colitis, human liver lesions, and xenic and axenic cultures. These particles are commonly arranged in rosettes and one or two rosette clusters are usually found surrounding a finely granular specialised area of the cytoplasm in thin sections of amoebae. Each cluster is about 1 μm in diameter and is composed of 9–30 cylindrical bodies. The bodies vary in size and may be up to 250 nm in length and 90 nm in width, surrounded by a 7 nm thick membrane. They tend to be bullet-shaped, although occasionally they appear rounded at both ends (Figure 4). The morphological similarity of the

---

[n]An EST for *E. dispar* profilin has also been identified (59).

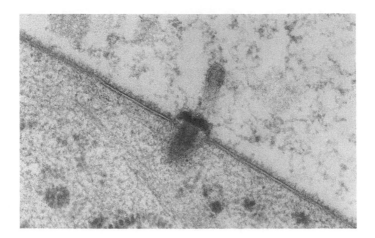

Figure 4. Transmission electron micrograph of a cryofixed and cryosubstituted *E. histolytica* trophozoite.

Bullet-shaped cylindrical bodies, morphologically similar to rhabdoviruses, can be observed apparently exiting the trophozoite through the plasma membrane by an as yet undescribed mechanism. The nature and biological significance of these particles remains unknown. Magnification X 166,000 (Courtesy of Dr. Arturo González-Robles).

cylindrical particles to rhabdoviruses and the cytochemical detection of a dense RNA-containing core in the rosette arrangements has led to speculation about their possible viral nature (127). There is, however, no conclusive evidence to date about their nature and biological significance. A number of morphologically distinct *E. histolytica* viruses were described in the 1970's and shown to have lytic capabilities (182). No recent studies have been published on these, however.

The plasma membrane

The plasma membrane of *E. histolytica* is approximately 10 nm thick and is covered by a uniform surface coat mainly composed of glycoproteins and lipophosphoglycans. The binding of the lectin concanavalin A (Con A) to the surface of the trophozoite induces rapid agglutination of the parasites. In contrast, *E. dispar* is markedly less susceptible to Con A agglutination (13). Recent studies with axenic cultures revealed a noticeably thinner surface coat in *E. dispar* when compared to *E. histolytica*, and a higher negative surface charge of the former as measured by microelectrophoresis (126). The differences in surface charge and agglutination with Con A between *E. dispar* and *E. histolytica* may be related to the clear-cut differences in the ultrastructure of the surface coat of both species. In actively motile trophozoites a thin layer of material is deposited on the substrate, leaving a trail with cytochemical properties similar to those of the surface coat (127).

Membrane lipids have been studied both in whole extracts of trophozoites (183) and in isolated plasma and internal membrane fractions (184). Cholesterol is enriched in the plasma membrane, consistent with previous reports in other types of cells. Phosphatidylethanolamine predominates over phosphatidylcholine in the plasma membrane, although the latter is the most abundant lipid in internal vesicles. An unusual phospholipid, ceramide aminoethyl phosphonate, has been demonstrated in internal vesicles, but is mostly concentrated in the plasma membrane, where it accounts for 35% of the total lipid content (184). This may have biological importance, since this compound is resistant to hydrolysis and may protect the parasite against the action of its own phospholipases.

Several surface molecules that mediate adhesion to cells or intestinal mucus are recognised by sera from patients with or cured of invasive amoebiasis. These include a 260 kDa galactose and N-acetyl-D-galactosamine inhibitable lectin which is a heterodimer of 170 kDa and 35 kDa subunits (155), a 220 kDa N-acetylglucosamine inhibitable lectin (185), a 125 kDa major surface peptide (186) and a 112 kDa surface adhesin (187). Antibodies raised against these proteins can partially inhibit adhesion to and phagocytosis of target cells in vitro, suggesting their participation in amoebic adherence. The 112 kDa adhesin appears to be formed through the association of two subunits, one with adhesin and the other with protease characteristics, encoded by adjacent genes (188). In addition, *E. histolytica* expresses a highly polymorphic lipophosphoglycan (LPG)-like molecules on its surface, which may also be involved in adhesion (189–194). There are two LPG-like molecules in *E. histolytica*, one of which has structural similarity to the well-described LPG from *Leishmania*, the other being a lipopeptidophosphoglycan (191). LPG-like molecules could not be demonstrated on the surface of *E. dispar* (192, 193), which is consistent with the differences in the surface coat of this species.

Among the enzymes identified in the plasma membrane of *E. histolytica* are a Ca^{2+} and other cation transporting-ATPases, phospholipase A, a neuraminidase, and a metallocollagenase thought to play an important role during tissue invasion (reviewed by Espinosa Cantellano and Martínez-Palomo (195)). One of the several cysteine proteases described (see above) has potent proteolytic activity and is located on the surface (196, 197). The gene for this enzyme is absent from *E. dispar* (42) which may partially explain the increased expression of cysteine protease genes in *E. histolytica* correlated with virulence. Finally, the surface localisation of an alcohol/aldehyde dehydrogenase, first reported as a 96 kDa amoebic antigen, has recently been confirmed (198).

A number of genes encoding members of the ABC transporter family, which includes multi-drug resistance (*mdr*) and P-glycoprotein genes, have been cloned from *E. histolytica* (199–201). The normal function of these proteins is not known but transcription of one of the *mdr* P-glycoprotein genes is elevated in emetine resistant cells (200). Active transport of calcium is normally mediated by Ca^{2+}-dependent ATPases. In general, Ca^{2+}-ATPases of the plasma membrane are distinct from the ones present in the ER. In *E. histolytica* two different Ca^{2+}-ATPase genes have been identified (56, 202) but their subcellular localisation is not clear. Apart from the above no genes encoding transport/permease proteins have been identified in *E. histolytica*.

Electron-dense granules (EDGs), known to contain collagenase, can be observed associated with the plasma membrane of *E. histolytica*. Following activation with collagen, there is a considerable increase in the number of these bodies, which are released from the parasite surface through a budding process. This Ca^{2+}-stimulated cytoskeleton-dependent process correlates with an increase in collagenolytic activity of the trophozoites and has thus been linked to tissue invasion by the parasite (203, 204). Purified EDGs have been shown to contain at least 25 polypeptides, some of which have protease activity (205), further supporting their involvement in amoebic pathogenesis.

Interaction of the trophozoite plasma membrane with specific ligands induces a dramatic redistribution of surface components that accumulate at the uroid and are later released into the medium. This capping of surface molecules, suggested as a mechanism for evasion of the humoral immune response, occurs through a sliding mechanism that involves both actin and myosin and is regulated by calmodulin and a myosin light chain kinase (206, 207).

Cell locomotion

Trophozoites in culture can be observed actively moving, constantly extending surface projections such as pseudopodia, lamellae, and phagocytic stomata. These are involved in ingestion of bacteria and other food particles but, during infection of the human host, they also allow the parasite to penetrate and invade tissues, and are thus important in pathogenesis. Although *E. histolytica* seems to have a simple cytoskeleton, understanding the cytoskeletal rearrangements that occur during locomotion and extension of surface projections has proven a difficult challenge, and these processes are still largely unknown.

Perhaps the most complex and dynamic assemblies of actin filaments are those involved in cell locomotion. Actin has been demonstrated to be a key participant in locomotion through the use of drugs that prevent polymerisation and depolymerisation of actin filaments. In order to exert a mechanical force, a contractile assembly must be anchored at one end to cell membranes. In mammalian cells, stress fibres terminate at specialised regions of the plasma membrane known as adhesion plaques, and locomotion involves at least three processes: (i) extension of a leading edge, (ii) attachment to the surface through adhesion plaques, and (iii) pulling forward of the remainder of the cell.

Actin polymerisation has been shown to occur during pseudopod extension in *E. histolytica* (207). Transient stabilisation of actin filaments could be achieved through ABP-120, an actin binding protein that cross-links polymerised actin filaments into networks in growing pseudopodia in *Dictyostelium discoideum* (208), and has also been identified in pseudopodia in *E. histolytica* (173, 209), as well as through the action of F-actin capping proteins (58). The motive force underlying cytoplasmic streaming in other eukaryotes is a Ca^{2+}-activated interaction between actin and myosin, similar to the one described in muscle contraction. No reports are available on the $[Ca^{2+}]_i$ fluctuations during pseudopod extension in *E. histolytica*, but myosin II has been shown to be present in leading lamellae (207).

Although no stress fibres have been described in *E. histolytica*, interaction of trophozoites with fibronectin (FN) and other extracellular matrix substrates induces the formation of adhesion plaques.[o] Recognition and binding to FN seems to involve a 37 kDa FN-binding protein (210) and a 140 kDa integrin-like protein (211, 212). Isolated amoebic adhesion plaques have been shown to be composed mainly of actin filaments (175). In addition, four actin binding proteins were also identified. One of them was vinculin, which had not been

---

[o]When first reported in *E. histolytica* these structures were referred to as 'adhesion plates'. As they have subsequently been shown to be equivalent to adhesion plaques in other eukaryotes, the latter name is used here.

previously described in *E. histolytica*. Vinculin has been proposed to link actin to an integral membrane component during anchoring of the cytoskeleton to the plasma membrane in mammalian cells. The presence of α-actinin in *E. histolytica* has been reported (171), and the identification of this gel-forming protein in adhesion plaques suggests a role in the stabilisation of actin filaments. Isolated amoebic adhesion plaques also contain tropomyosin, which has not been reported in adhesion plaques in other eukaryotes but has been identified in stress fibres. In muscle cells, this rod-shaped, cofilamentous protein sterically blocks the interaction of actin and myosin, but shifts its position when the level of Ca^{2+} is raised (probably in response to a change in shape of the troponin molecules to which it is bound), thus allowing contraction to take place. As will be seen below, adhesion of *E. histolytica* trophozoites to FN induces a sustained rise of $[Ca^{2+}]_i$. It could be speculated that tropomyosin in adhesion plaques also regulates interaction of actin and myosin II, both shown to be present in these specialised structures. Finally, an unexpected finding in the isolated amoebic adhesion plaques was the presence of myosin I, a member of a family of unconventional myosins that have been related to the intracellular transport of vesicles, phagocytosis, pinocytosis and pseudopod extension (176, 213). Its function in adhesion plaques remains to be determined.

Amoebic adhesion plaques seem to be important not only in adhesion and locomotion of the parasite, but also in the degradation of extracellular matrix (ECM) components. This is supported by the detection of several protease activities in isolated adhesion plaques (175). The molecular weights of the activities identified in gelatin-containing SDS gels are similar to the 27–29 kDa and 56 kDa cysteine proteases, known to degrade FN and other ECM proteins (96, 110), and the 70 kDa membrane-associated protease (196).

The third process in cell motility, pulling forward of the remainder of the cell, is still obscure in *E. histolytica*. During locomotion, amoebae move towards the pseudopod, while leaving a trailing uroid. Actin and myosin II have been identified in the uroid (206), but no other regulatory proteins have been reported. In *D. dictyostelium* myosin II participates in detachment from the substratum and retraction of the cell (214).

Signal Transduction

The most mysterious aspect of locomotion is related to its control. Only recently have signalling pathways in *E. histolytica* started to be explored, but much is still unknown. In mammalian cells, several kinases have been reported to act as signal transducers of the initial ligand-receptor interaction, by phosphorylating themselves and other specific substrates, and activating second messengers such as Ca^{2+}, cyclic AMP and small GTP-binding proteins.

There is evidence to suggest that *E. histolytica* has an extensive signal transduction system though the factors that initiate these signals are not very well characterised. Many cell surface receptors, such as the 170 kDa Gal/GalNAc lectin, laminin receptor (56) and a homologue of the leukocyte adhesion molecule LECAM3 (57), could in principle initiate signalling after interaction with molecules present on the surface of bacteria and epithelial cells or extracellular matrix proteins. Transduction of signals may be through heterotrimeric G proteins (215) for which a gene encoding the β-chain has been found (57).

A number of genes encoding different protein kinases, including GTPases and multifunctional 14-3-3 kinases, have been identified in both *E. histolytica* and *E. dispar* (56, 59, 216–219). Homologues of protein phosphatases and tyrosine protein phosphatase have been identified in *E. dispar* (59) and *E. histolytica* (58), respectively, suggesting that *Entamoeba* may have signalling pathways that are quite similar to other eukaryotes. The functional details of the signalling pathways are not clear as yet as the target molecules for the kinases and phosphatases are not known.

Calcium is also an important molecule in cellular signal transduction system and can be released from internal stores by a mechanism based on inositol triphosphate (IP_3) receptor activation (220). Although biochemical evidence for the presence of a Ca^{2+}/calmodulin pathway has been reported (221) no calmodulin gene has yet been identified. Both *E. histolytica* and *E. dispar* may have a novel calcium signal transduction system, as a calcium binding protein of the calmodulin family, but with no specific homology to any known protein, has been discovered in these species (222, 223).

The most complete study to date of signal transduction in *E. histolytica* concerns the interaction of trophozoites with ECM components, which induces structural and metabolic changes that suggest the activation of intracellular pathways described in other eukaryotic cells (175, 224–227). As stated above, interaction of *E. histolytica* with FN induces a marked reorganisation of the actin cytoskeleton with the formation of adhesion plaques. It has been shown that FN binding transduces information into the trophozoites, activating a protein kinase C (PKC) pathway with the production of IP_3 and the phosphorylation of several proteins, probably including PKC itself. Activation of PKC through binding of FN or direct stimulation with phorbol myristate acetate shows a direct relationship with actin polymerisation and assembly of various actin binding proteins in the adhesion plaques. Moreover, activated PKC is translated to the cytoskeleton fraction during stimulation (227). Although the targets of PKC have not been identified, its activation sheds some light on one signalling pathway in the parasite.

A second signalling pathway seems to occur via a focal adhesion kinase, pp125^{FAK}, which is part of a complex of proteins known to be phosphotyrosine substrates for the *src* family of tyrosine kinases. pp125^{FAK} has been identified by a chicken anti-pp125^{FAK} antibody in immunoblots of isolated amoebic adhesion plaques induced by FN, suggesting a role of this signal transducer in the formation of adhesion plaques (175). Moreover, adhesion of *E. histolytica* trophozoites to collagen induces phosphorylation of several proteins, one of which has been identified as pp125^{FAK} by monoclonal antibodies, further suggesting its participation in signal transduction (226). It has been suggested that activation of pp125^{FAK} might initiate a signal transduction pathway that activates the mitogen-activated protein kinase (MAPK) cascade, allowing the flow of information from the ECM to the cell interior. This is supported by the identification of p42^{MAPK} in tyrosine phosphorylated polypeptides induced by collagen-stimulated trophozoites (226).

Incubation of trophozoites with FN produces a sustained rise in [Ca^{2+}]$_i$ levels, which promotes stabilisation of adhesion plaques and focal contacts by shifting soluble, monomeric G-actin to the polymerised F-actin configuration. External Ca^{2+} influx has been shown to be responsible for the increased [Ca^{2+}]$_i$ levels, since cytoplasmic Ca^{2+} stores are rapidly depleted (224). The role of Ca^{2+} remains to be established, but its absence results in poor adhesion of trophozoites, suggesting at least its participation in actin organisation. Since tropomyosin has been identified in isolated adhesion plaques, it is tempting to speculate that this rod-shaped protein might regulate actin-myosin interaction, as occurs in muscle cells, where increased Ca^{2+} levels induce a conformational change in troponin that shifts the position of tropomyosin, thus allowing the interaction between actin and myosin.

Recent studies indicate that actin organisation might have different levels of regulation, namely through changes in actin gene expression and the balance between the G-actin and F-actin configurations. Treatment of *E. histolytica* trophozoites with drugs known to increase cytoplasmic cyclic AMP levels (forskolin and dibutyryl cyclic AMP) or to activate PKC (phorbol myristate acetate) produces a shift in the actin equilibrium to the F-actin form, which in turn increases actin mRNA levels in these cells (225). This suggests an actin-feedback regulatory mechanism, previously described in other cells, where the protein product and the configuration of the microfilaments could directly regulate actin gene expression (225). Evidence for another regulatory mechanism in actin organisation is provided by the isolation and cDNA cloning of the *E. histolytica* profilin basic isoform (178). Profilin has been shown in other systems to act as a buffer in actin organisation by inhibiting or promoting actin filament formation, depending on the conditions.

Genome Structure

Recent studies have started to reveal the structure and organisation of the *E. histolytica* genome. However, there is still uncertainty surrounding the exact ploidy, DNA content of the nucleus and the presence of cytoplasmic DNA, among other features.

Linear DNA

It has been estimated that the *E. histolytica* DNA content is 0.24 picogrammes per cell (138). If the ploidy of *E. histolytica* is indeed 4n (see above) the total haploid genome size would be about 50 million base-pairs (Mb). There was some initial difficulty in obtaining well resolved separations of *E. histolytica* chromosomal sized-DNA using Pulsed Field Gel Electrophoresis (PFGE; among others (228–230)), but two groups have recently reported success (122, 231). The electrophoretic karyotype of *E. histolytica* has been determined using PFGE and the size of the haploid genome estimated to be about 20 Mb, which is slightly smaller than many parasitic protozoan genomes (122). There are about 31–35 chromosomes ranging in size from 0.3 to 2.2 Mb, depending on the isolate used for analysis, and 14 linkage groups each with a ploidy of up to 4 (122).

The structure and organisation of *E. histolytica* chromosomes is not yet clear, but like other protozoan parasites *E. histolytica* exhibits considerable genomic plasticity, as shown by the fact that homologous chromosomes of different isolates show distinct size variation. This is further complicated by observed size differences among allelic chromosomes within a given isolate (122, 231). Whether size variation observed in *E. histolytica* is due to extensive amplification and deletion of telomeric and/or subtelomeric repeats, as observed for other protozoan parasites, remains to be investigated. Unfortunately, there is still no information about the structure of the

E. histolytica telomere or whether chromosomal ends have a different organisation. The hybridisation of certain PFGE DNA bands to heterologous telomeric DNA probes is suggestive but there is as yet no proof that the probe is detecting telomeres in *E. histolytica* (230).

There are several classes of dispersed and tandemly repeated DNAs in *E. histolytica* (232–235). The functions of these sequence elements have not yet been described.

Circular and Cytoplasmic DNAs

The *E. histolytica* ribosomal RNA genes (rDNA) are carried on circular DNA molecules. This was reported independently by two groups (236, 237). The complete sequence of one rDNA circle has been published (238, 239). It measures 24.5 kilobasepairs (kb) in length and carries two copies of the ribosomal RNA cistron as an inverted repeat. It encodes the small, large and 5.8S rRNAs but not the 5S rRNA. No proteins are encoded. Several classes of tandemly repeated DNAs are present, some of which are interrelated and one of which is transcribed. Certain regions of the plasmid are unstable in that length variation due to changes in the number of repeat units occurs quite frequently (240, 241). The plasmid structure just described is not universal, however. In a few isolates, only one rDNA cistron is present and certain repeated DNA classes are missing also (238, 242). The single rDNA cistron structure was also found in one isolate of *E. moshkovskii*, but the structure in other *Entamoeba* species remains to be determined. As stated earlier, in situ hybridisation indicates that the rDNA is found in the periphery of the nucleus (128).

In addition to the 24.5 kb rDNA circles, two groups have reported the presence of less abundant nuclear DNA circles in different size classes of ca. 5 kb, 12 kb and 50 kb in length (228, 243). The coding potential, structure and complexity of these molecules has not been studied. The presence and abundance of these several size classes of circular DNAs may in part be responsible for the early reports of difficulty in obtaining well resolved separations of *E. histolytica* DNA in PFGE. Several classes of dispersed and tandemly repeated DNAs have been described that are not associated with the rDNA circle (232–235).

One group recently has published reports purporting to demonstrate the existence of cytoplasmic DNA in *E. histolytica*, including cytoplasmic rDNA (244, 245). This requires independent confirmation as it is in conflict with several earlier published reports. Previously, metabolic labelling with thymidine (246), staining with DNA-binding dyes (138) and in situ hybridisation with rDNA (128) all failed to detect cytoplasmic DNA, in contrast to the most recent reports. The same group (245) also found circular DNAs smaller than those reported by other authors (228, 243).

Transcription, Translation and Replication

The mechanism of transcription is poorly understood in *E. histolytica* and EST analysis has not to date yielded any new information. Except for a TATA-box binding protein (TBP) gene (247) no others encoding any protein involved in transcription have been reported. A few *E. histolytica* and *E. dispar* genes have introns (140, 248–250); these are shorter than in most other eukaryotes. The mRNA splicing machinery must be present for processing of these pre-mRNAs. This is supported by the isolation of the gene encoding U6 small nuclear RNA from *E. histolytica* (251). Transcription does not show the same drug sensitivity seen in most other eukaryotes (252). More details of gene structure, promoter analysis and transfection will be found in another chapter.

A number of genes encoding proteins involved in the assembly of ribosomes and the translational apparatus have been cloned from *E. histolytica* and *E. dispar*. So far, 39 large subunit ribosomal proteins (of the 49 present in an average eukaryote) and 27 small subunit ribosomal proteins (of the 33 present in an average eukaryote) have been identified (56–59). The proteins show a high degree of similarity to homologues from other eukaryotic organisms. Apart from ribosomal proteins, homologues of eIF5A (of *E. dispar* (59)) and eIF2 (of *E. histolytica* (56)), two key molecules in eukaryotic translation initiation, have also been identified. eIF5A is the only protein known to contain the post-translationally modified amino acid deoxyhypusine. This modification has an important role in translation and cell growth (253). An EST encoding the enzyme deoxyhypusine synthase has been isolated from *E. dispar* (59) suggesting that the modification is also present in this organism. Elongation factors EF-1α (254) and EF-2 (255) have also been characterised (56–59).

Small subunit, 5.8S, and large subunit rRNA equivalents have been characterised extensively in *E. histolytica* (238, 256, 257), and the 5.8S rRNA genes of *E. dispar* (257, 258), *E. moshkovskii* (259) and *E. invadens* (256, 258), and the small subunit genes of numerous species (8, 260–262) have also been sequenced. When compared to ribosomal RNAs of other organisms the

Entamoeba rRNAs have the features characteristic of all eukaryotes. So far, 5S rRNA genes have not been isolated from any species of *Entamoeba* and only one tRNA gene sequence has been reported, from *E. histolytica* (263).

There is very little information available on the mechanism of DNA replication in *E. histolytica*. Only one relevant gene, encoding a homologue of the yeast 'mini chromosome maintenance' gene *mcm3*, has been identified so far (264). This protein is much smaller than its homologues in other eukaryotes, which have been implicated in DNA replication. In the absence of any other information it is difficult to predict the function of this protein in *E. histolytica*. DNA polymerase activity has been detected in both *E. histolytica* and *E. invadens* (265–267). Based on sensitivity to drugs such as aphidicolin, it appears that this enzyme may belong to the alpha family of DNA polymerases. Replication has only been studied directly in the case of the rDNA circle. Extensive analysis using two dimensional gel electrophoresis and electron microscopy revealed that initiation of replication is promiscuous (268), although some sites are preferred over others. Establishing the generality of this observation and the nature of the origins of replication will require a significant amount of additional work.

Polyadenylated nontranslatable RNAs

Four different classes of polyadenylated RNAs lacking significant protein-encoding capacity (IE, *Tr*, UEE1, ehapt1) have been characterised in *E. histolytica* (for a review see Ref. 269). Together they constitute the most abundant poly A-containing RNAs in *E. histolytica* (58). It does not appear that any post-transcriptional sequence editing is taking place in these transcripts as cDNA and genomic sequences are identical. Except for *Tr*, which is present on the ribosomal episome (see above), these transcripts are encoded by multicopy chromosomal genes and show considerable sequence heterogeneity within each class.

The transcript *Tr* is encoded in the rDNA plasmid of many strains of *E. histolytica* and so far has not been found in any other species (239). UEE1 was identified during EST analysis of *E. dispar* (59) and by database search two ESTs of *E. histolytica* were also found which showed significant sequence identity with UEE1. It is present in at least four copies per haploid genome equivalent and represents about 8% of all the cDNAs of *E. dispar*. Not all UEE1s are identical and they display about 2–14% sequence divergence from each other. The first two members of IE family of sequences were described seven years ago (233) and consisted of a genomic clone and a very similar but not quite identical sequence present in a cDNA library. In all, partial or nearly complete sequences of cDNAs for about 20 RNA transcripts are now known and thought to be dispersed throughout the genome with the majority present in intergenic regions. The fourth class of these novel RNAs, ehapt1, was also identified during EST analysis of *E. histolytica* HM-1:IMSS (58).

The functions of these transcripts are still unknown. They may function as RNA molecules as suggested by presence of extensive secondary structures. So far there are no data to offer any idea about the function of these molecules. It has been speculated that these may be involved in regulation of transcription. To our knowledge presence of such transcripts has not been yet been reported from other protozoa.

Genetic variation

Isoenzymes

Sargeaunt and colleagues described over twenty zymodemes that are now divided between *E. histolytica* and *E. dispar* (15). However, it is not clear how many of these are real. Blanc and Sargeaunt (270) first indicated that the presence of some isoenzyme bands was dependent on the specific culture conditions, namely the amount of starch in the medium. Subsequently, Jackson's group (271) and Diamond's group (273) independently showed that upon axenisation the 'secondary' isoenzyme bands used to define most of the *E. histolytica* zymodemes disappeared.[p] Diamond's group (273) has further shown that, in at least some cases, these 'secondary' isoenzyme bands are likely to be of bacterial rather than amoebal origin. The current number of 'principal' (272) zymodemes (those that are found in axenic cultures) in *E. histolytica* is only three, those known as zymodemes II, XIV and XIX, and in *E. dispar* only one (zymodeme I).

Isoenzymes were also used to study potential genetic exchange in *E. histolytica* (274, 275) but, in view of the above mentioned doubts over zymodeme interpretation, this work is in need of careful verification. A recent report on the isolation from humans of an *E. histolytica* in which the isoenzyme pattern is suggested to be the result of genetic exchange must likewise be treated with caution (276).

---

[p]This is also true of *E. dispar* in axenic culture (41).

DNA

As mentioned above, some repeated DNAs carried on the rDNA circles exhibit length variation due to changes in the numbers of repetitive elements, presumably due to intra- or inter-molecular recombination (240, 241). While this occurred quite rapidly within one cloned isolate, the observed changes involved only one of the repeated DNAs. A second repeat region located on the ribosomal plasmid (*Tr*, above, also known as SSG) also exhibits length variation but in this case the changes are much less frequent so that variation is only detected when different isolates of *E. histolytica* are compared (277).

Protein encoding genes can also exhibit internally repeated structures — this is most common in but not exclusive to surface antigens. In *E. histolytica*, two genes have been described that exhibit significant intraspecific genetic variation. Both the number and the sequence of the repeats are involved and the homologous genes in *E. dispar* show a similar pattern of variation. The first report involved the serine-rich *E. histolytica* protein (277). This protein contains two types of repeats of eight and twelve amino acids in length. The two repeats are themselves related in sequence. The variation appears to be relatively stable, being unaffected by long term cultivation or axenisation, for example (277). The second gene to exhibit variation was that encoding chitinase, where near the amino terminus of the protein there are repeats that vary in both length and sequence among isolates (278). These polymorphic markers have the potential to be used in tracking infection transmission. The existence of polymorphism among alleles of the same gene has also been noted in ESTs (58).

There is also chromosomal size polymorphism in *E. histolytica*. Genes thought to be present in a single copy were found to hybridise to multiple bands in PFGE (122, 231). Though linkage groups were found to be conserved the sizes of the allelic chromosomes within strains and homologous chromosomes between strains were quite different. Though there is little experimental data so far it appears that the variation may be due to deletion or expansion of telomeric or subtelomeric repeated sequences.

Conclusions

While still unique in a number of ways, it is becoming clear that *E. histolytica* is not as different from other eukaryotes as was initially thought. Recent studies show that it does have most of the biochemical and cellular features of other eukaryotic cells and that its novel features may be due in large part to adaptation to the gut environment. It is also clear that there remain major gaps in our understanding of the basic biology of the organism. We hope that this overview of the biology of *Entamoeba histolytica* rapidly becomes out of date!

Acknowledgements

The authors wish to thank Drs. Bibiana Chávez and Arturo González Robles for their generous gift of unpublished electron micrographs. AB thanks Dr. Sudha Bhattacharya for helpful comments and MEC thanks Drs. Adolfo Martínez-Palomo and Isaura Meza for critical reading of the cell biology sections of the manuscript.

References

1. Lösch F (1875). *Virchow's Archiv* **65**: 196.
2. Schaudinn F (1903). *Arbeit. Kaiserlichen Gesundheitsamte* **19**: 547.
3. Dobell C (1919) *The amoebae living in man. A zoological monograph* (J. Bale, Sons, and Danielson, London).
4. von Prowazek S (1912). *Arch. Protistenk.* **26**: 241.
5. Burrows RB (1957). *Am. J. Hyg.* **65**: 172.
6. Goldman M, *et al.* (1960). *Exp. Parasitol.* **10**: 366.
7. Clark CG and Diamond LS (1997). *J. Euk. Microbiol.* **44**: 142.
8. Silberman JD, *et al.* (1999). *Mol. Biol. Evol.* (In Press).
9. Brumpt E (1925). *Bull. Acad. Méd. (Paris)* **94**: 943.
10. Walker EL and Sellards AW (1913). *Phillipine J. Sci. B Trop. Med.* **8**: 253.
11. Simic T (1931). *Ann. Parasitol. Hum. Comp.* **9**: 385.
12. Simic T (1931). *Ann. Parasitol. Hum. Comp.* **9**: 497.
13. Martínez-Palomo A, *et al.* (1973). *Nature New Biol.* **245**: 186.
14. Sargeaunt PG, *et al.* (1978). *Trans. R. Soc. Trop. Med. Hyg.* **72**: 519.
15. Sargeaunt PG (1987). *Parasitol. Today* **3**: 40.
16. Sargeaunt PG, *et al.* (1982). *Arch. Invest. Méd. (Méx.)* **13 (suppl 3)**: 89.
17. Strachan WD, *et al.* (1988). *Lancet* **i**: 561.
18. Tannich E, *et al.* (1989). *Proc. Natl. Acad. Sci. USA* **86**: 5118.
19. Diamond LS and Clark CG (1993). *J. Euk. Microbiol.* **40**: 340.
20. Anonymous (1997). *Bull. Wld. Hlth. Org.* **75**: 291.

21. Mirelman D, *et al.* (1986). *Exp. Parasitol.* **62**: 142.
22. Mirelman D, *et al.* (1986). *Infect. Immun.* **54**: 827.
23. Vrchotová N, *et al.* (1993). *Ann. Parasitol. Hum. Comp.* **68**: 67.
24. Vargas MA and Orozco E (1993). *Parasitol. Res.* **79**: 353.
25. Mukherjee RM, *et al.* (1993). *Trans. R. Soc. Trop. Med. Hyg.* **87**: 490.
26. Andrews BJ, *et al.* (1990). *Trans. R. Soc. Trop. Med. Hyg.* **84**: 63.
27. Clark CG and Diamond LS (1993). *Exp. Parasitol.* **77**: 456.
28. Tshalaia LE (1941). *Med. Parazit. (Moscow)* **10**: 244.
29. Richards CS, *et al.* (1966). *Am. J. Trop. Med. Hyg.* **15**: 648.
30. Beaver PC, *et al.* (1956). *Am. J. Trop. Med. Hyg.* **5**: 1015.
31. Beaver PC, *et al.* (1956). *Am. J. Trop. Med. Hyg.* **5**: 1000.
32. Clark CG and Diamond LS (1991). *Mol. Biochem. Parasitol.* **46**: 11.
33. Sargeaunt PG, *et al.* (1992). *Trans. R. Soc. Trop. Med. Hyg.* **86**: 633.
34. Chacín-Bonilla L (1992). *Trans. R. Soc. Trop. Med. Hyg.* **86**: 634.
35. Clark CG and Diamond LS (1992). *Am. J. Trop. Med. Hyg.* **46**: 158.
36. Vogel P, *et al.* (1996). *Am. J. Trop. Med. Hyg.* **55**: 595.
37. Dobell C (1938). *Parasitology* **30**: 195.
38. Bakker-Grunwald T and Wöstmann C (1993). *Parasitol. Today* **9**: 27.
39. Meza I (1992). *Arch. Med. Res.* **23**: 1.
40. Blanc DS (1992). *J. Protozool.* **39**: 471.
41. Clark CG (1995). *J. Euk. Microbiol.* **42**: 590.
42. Bruchhaus I, *et al.* (1996). *Mol. Microbiol.* **22**: 255.
43. Willhoeft U, *et al.* (1999). *Parasitol. Res.* **85**: 787.
44. Clark CG (1995). *Trop. Dis. Bull.* **92**: R147.
45. Boeck WC and Drbohlav J (1925). *Amer. J. Hyg.* **5**: 371.
46. Diamond LS (1983). *In vitro cultivation of protozoan parasites*, ed. Jensen JB (CRC Press, Boca Raton, FL) 67.
47. Robinson GL (1968). *Trans. R. Soc. Trop. Med. Hyg.* **62**: 285.
48. Diamond LS (1982). *J. Parasitol.* **68**: 958.
49. Diamond LS (1961). *Science* **134**: 336.
50. Diamond LS (1968). *J. Parasitol.* **54**: 715.
51. Diamond LS (1968). *J. Parasitol.* **54**: 1047.
52. Diamond LS, *et al.* (1978). *Trans. R. Soc. Trop. Med. Hyg.* **72**: 431.
53. Kobayashi S, *et al.* (1998). *J. Euk. Microbiol.* **45**: 3S.
54. Diamond LS, *et al.* (1995). *J. Euk. Microbiol.* **42**: 277.
55. Reeves RE (1984). *Adv. Parasitol.* **23**: 105.
56. Azam A, *et al.* (1996). *Gene* **181**: 113.
57. Tanaka T, *et al.* (1997). *Biochem. Biophys. Res. Commun.* **236**: 611.
58. Willhoeft U, *et al.* (1999). *Protist* **150**: 61.

59. Sharma R, *et al.* (1999). *Mol. Biochem. Parasitol.* **99**: 279.
60. Lo H and Reeves RE (1980). *Mol. Biochem. Parasitol.* **2**: 23.
61. Bruchhaus I, *et al.* (1998). *Biochem. J.* **330**: 1217.
62. Bruchhaus I and Tannich E (1994). *Mol. Biochem. Parasitol.* **67**: 281.
63. Tannich E, *et al.* (1991). *Mol. Biochem. Parasitol.* **49**: 61.
64. Fahey RC, *et al.* (1984). *Science* **224**: 70.
65. Ariyanayagam MR and Fairlamb AH (1999). *Mol. Biochem. Parasitol.* **103**: 61
66. Bruchhaus I, *et al.* (1997). *Biochem. J.* **326**: 785.
67. Poole LB, *et al.* (1997). *Free Radical Biol. Med.* **23**: 955.
68. Nozaki T, *et al.* (1998). *Mol. Biochem. Parasitol.* **97**: 33.
69. Nozaki T (1999). (Unpublished) GenBank Accession Numbers: AB013399, AB023954.
70. Diamond LS and Cunnick CC (1991). *J. Protozool.* **38**: 211.
71. Bakker-Grunwald T, *et al.* (1995). *J. Euk. Microbiol.* **42**: 346.
72. Rosenthal B, *et al.* (1997). *J. Bacteriol.* **179**: 3736.
73. Ortner S, *et al.* (1997). *Mol. Biochem. Parasitol.* **90**: 121.
74. Werries E and Müller F (1986). *Mol. Biochem. Parasitol.* **18**: 211.
75. Ortner S, *et al.* (1997). *Mol. Biochem. Parasitol.* **86**: 85.
76. Huang M, *et al.* (1995). *Biochim. Biophys. Acta* **1260**: 215.
77. Bruchhaus I, *et al.* (1996). *Biochem. J.* **316**: 57.
78. Deng Z, *et al.* (1998). *Biochem. J.* **329**: 659.
79. Landa A, *et al.* (1997). *Eur. J. Biochem.* **247**: 348.
80. Beanan MJ and Bailey GB (1995). *Mol. Biochem. Parasitol.* **69**: 119.
81. Hidalgo ME, *et al.* (1997). *FEMS Microbiol. Letts.* **148**: 123.
82. Bruchhaus I and Tannich E (1993). *Mol. Biochem. Parasitol.* **62**: 153.
83. Saavedra-Lira E and Pérez-Montfort R (1994). *Gene* **142**: 249.
84. Huber M, *et al.* (1988). *Mol. Biochem. Parasitol.* **31**: 27.
85. Rodríguez MA, *et al.* (1996). *Mol. Biochem. Parasitol.* **78**: 273.
86. Thammapalerd N, *et al.* (1996). *S. E. Asian J. Trop. Med. Publ. Hlth.* **27**: 63.
87. Samuelson J (1995). (Unpublished) GenBank Accession Number: U30611.
88. Bruchhaus I and Tannich E (1994). *Biochem. J.* **303**: 743.
89. Yang W, *et al.* (1994). *Mol. Biochem. Parasitol.* **64**: 253.
90. Rodríguez MA, *et al.* (1996). *Biochim. Biophys. Acta* **1306**: 23.
91. Kimura A, *et al.* (1996). *Clin. Diagn. Lab. Immunol.* **3**: 270.
92. Kumar A, *et al.* (1992). *Proc. Natl. Acad. Sci. USA* **89**: 10188.
93. Rodríguez MA, *et al.* (1998). *Microb. Pathogenesis* **25**: 1.

94. Weinbach EC and Diamond LS (1974). *Exp. Parasitol.* **35**: 232.
95. Ellis JE, *et al.* (1994). *Mol. Biochem. Parasitol.* **65**: 213.
96. Weinbach EC, *et al.* (1976). *Proc. of the Int. Conf. on Amebiasis*, eds. Sepúlveda B and Diamond LS (IMSS, Mexico City, Mexico) 190.
97. Harlow DR, *et al.* (1976). *Comp. Biochem. Physiol. [B]* **53**: 141.
98. Yu Y and Samuelson J (1994). *Mol. Biochem. Parasitol.* **68**: 323.
99. Clark CG and Roger AJ (1995). *Proc. Natl. Acad. Sci. USA* **92**: 6518.
100. Vargas-Villareal J, *et al.* (1995). *Parasitol. Res.* **81**: 320.
101. Vargas-Villareal J, *et al.* (1998). *Parasitol. Res.* **84**: 310.
102. Luján HD and Diamond LS (1997). *Arch. Med. Res.* **28 (suppl.)**: S96. (Abstract)
103. Lohia A, *et al.* (1999). *Mol. Biochem. Parasitol.* **98**: 67.
104. Samuelson J and Field J (1999). (Unpublished) GenBank Accession Number: AF118848.
105. Vargas-Rodríguez L, *et al.* (1998). *Int. J. Parasitol.* **28**: 1333.
106. Villagómez-Castro JC, *et al.* (1998). *Exp. Parasitol.* **88**: 111.
107. Keene WE, *et al.* (1990). *Exp. Parasitol.* **71**: 199.
108. Keene WE, *et al.* (1986). *J. Exp. Med.* **163**: 536.
109. Luaces AL and Barret AJ (1988). *Biochem. J.* **250**: 903.
110. Montfort I, *et al.* (1993). *J. Parasitol.* **79**: 98.
111. Scholze H, *et al.* (1992). *Arch. Med. Res.* **23**: 105.
112. Lushbaugh WB, *et al.* (1985). *Exp. Parasitol.* **59**: 328.
113. Sharma M, *et al.* (1996). *Exp. Parasitol.* **84**: 84.
114. Scholze H, *et al.* (1996). *J. Biol. Chem.* **271**: 6212.
115. Wöstmann C, *et al.* (1992). *FEBS Letts.* **308**: 54.
116. Ramos MA, *et al.* (1997). *Mol. Biochem. Parasitol.* **84**: 131.
117. Hellberg A, *et al.* (1999). *Parasitol. Res.* **85**: 417.
118. Wöstmann C, *et al.* (1996). *Mol. Biochem. Parasitol.* **82**: 81.
119. Dobell C (1928). *Parasitology* **20**: 357.
120. Hegner R, *et al.* (1932). *Am. J. Hyg.* **15**: 394.
121. Sirijintakarn P and Bailey GB (1980). *Arch. Invest. Méd. (Méx.)* **11**: 3.
122. Willhoeft U and Tannich E (1999). *Mol. Biochem. Parasitol.* **99**: 41.
123. Eichinger D (1997). *BioEssays* **19**: 633.
124. de la Vega H, *et al.* (1997). *Mol. Biochem. Parasitol.* **85**: 139.
125. Walderich B, *et al.* (1998). *Am. J. Trop. Med. Hyg.* **59**: 342.
126. Espinosa-Cantellano M, *et al.* (1998). *J. Euk. Microbiol.* **45**: 265.
127. Martínez-Palomo A (1982). *The biology of Entamoeba histolytica* (John Wiley & Sons, Chichester).
128. Zurita M, *et al.* (1991). *Mol. Microbiol.* **5**: 1843.

129. Födinger M, *et al.* (1993). *Mol. Biochem. Parasitol.* **59**: 315.
130. Binder M, *et al.* (1995). *Mol. Biochem. Parasitol.* **71**: 243.
131. Scharfetter JK, *et al.* (1997). *Arch. Med. Res.* **28 (suppl.)**: S14. (Abstract)
132. Sánchez LB, *et al.* (1994). *Mol. Biochem. Parasitol.* **67**: 137.
133. Torres-Guerrero H, *et al.* (1991). *Mol. Biochem. Parasitol.* **45**: 121.
134. González-Robles A (1997). (Unpublished).
135. Ray SS, *et al.* (1997). *Mol. Biochem. Parasitol.* **90**: 331.
136. Argüello C, *et al.* (1992). *Arch. Med. Res.* **23**: 77.
137. Gómez-Conde E, *et al.* (1998). *Exp. Parasitol.* **89**: 122.
138. Dvorak JA, *et al.* (1995). *J. Euk. Microbiol.* **42**: 610.
139. Vohra H, *et al.* (1998). *Parasitol. Res.* **84**: 835.
140. Lohia A and Samuelson J (1993). *Gene* **127**: 203.
141. Shen P-S, *et al.* (1994). *Mol. Biochem. Parasitol.* **64**: 111.
142. Lohia A and Samuelson J (1994). *Biochim. Biophys. Acta* **1222**: 122.
143. Lohia A and Samuelson J (1993). *Mol. Biochem. Parasitol.* **58**: 177.
144. Martínez-Palomo A (1986) *Amebiasis*, ed. Martínez-Palomo A (Elsevier, Amsterdam) 12.
145. Beanan MJ and Bailey GB (1995). *J. Euk. Microbiol.* **42**: 632.
146. Temesvari LA, *et al.* (1999). *Mol. Biochem. Parasitol.* **103**: 225
147. Löhden-Bendinger U and Bakker-Grunwald T (1990). *Z. Naturforsch.* **45c**: 229.
148. Yi Y and Samuelson J (1994). *Mol. Biochem. Parasitol.* **66**: 165.
149. Descoteaux S, *et al.* (1994). *Infect. Immun.* **62**: 3572.
150. Ghosh SK and Samuelson J (1997). *Infect. Immun.* **65**: 4243.
151. Jacobs T and Leippe M (1995). *Eur. J. Biochem.* **231**: 831.
152. Leippe M, *et al.* (1994). *Mol. Microbiol.* **14**: 895.
153. Nickel R, *et al.* (1998). *FEBS Letts.* **437**: 153.
154. Ramos MA, *et al.* (1997). *Mol. Biochem. Parasitol.* **88**: 225.
155. Petri Jr WA (1996). *J. Investig. Med.* **44**: 24.
156. McCoy JJ, *et al.* (1993). *J. Biol. Chem.* **268**: 24223.
157. Kuzna-Grygiel W (1994). *Acta Protozool.* **33**: 233.
158. Mazzuco A, *et al.* (1997). *Micron* **28**: 241.
159. Kimura A, *et al.* (1997). *Arch. Med. Res.* **28 (suppl.)**: S76. (Abstract)
160. Monnat J, *et al.* (1997). *FEBS Letts.* **418**: 357.
161. Sánchez-López R, *et al.* (1998). *Mol. Biochem. Parasitol.* **92**: 355.
162. Ghosh SK, *et al.* (1999). *Infect. Immun.* **67**: 3073.
163. Bakatselou C and Clark CG (1999). (Unpublished).
164. Roger AJ, *et al.* (1998). *Proc. Natl. Acad. Sci. USA* **95**: 229.
165. Mai Z, *et al.* (1999). *Mol. Cell. Biol.* **19**: 2198.

166. Tovar J, *et al.* (1999). *Mol. Microbiol.* **32**: 1013.
167. Edman U, *et al.* (1987). *Proc. Natl. Acad. Sci. USA* **84**: 3024.
168. Huber M, *et al.* (1987). *Mol. Biochem. Parasitol.* **24**: 227.
169. Meza I, *et al.* (1983). *J. Biol. Chem.* **258**: 3936.
170. Sussman DJ, *et al.* (1984). *J. Biol. Chem.* **259**: 7349.
171. Bailey GB, *et al.* (1992). *Arch. Med. Res.* **23**: 129.
172. Rahim Z, *et al.* (1993). *Infect. Immun.* **61**: 1048.
173. Vargas M, *et al.* (1996). *Mol. Microbiol.* **22**: 849.
174. Arhets P, *et al.* (1998). *Mol. Biol. Cell* **8**: 1547.
175. Vázquez J, *et al.* (1995). *Cell Motil. Cytoskel.* **32**: 37.
176. Vargas MA, *et al.* (1997). *Mol. Biochem. Parasitol.* **86**: 61.
177. Voigt H, *et al.* (1999). *J. Cell Sci.* **112**: 1191.
178. Binder M, *et al.* (1995). *Eur. J. Biochem.* **233**: 976.
179. González-Robles A and Martínez-Palomo A (1992). *Arch. Med. Res.* **23**: 73.
180. Katiyar SK and Edlind TD (1996). *J. Euk. Microbiol.* **43**: 31.
181. Sánchez MA, *et al.* (1994). *Gene* **146**: 239.
182. Diamond LS and Mattern CFT (1976). *Adv. Virus Res.* **20**: 87.
183. Cerbón J and Flores J (1981). *Comp. Biochem. Physiol. [B]* **69**: 487.
184. Aley SB, *et al.* (1980). *J. Exp. Med.* **152**: 397.
185. Rosales-Encina JL, *et al.* (1987). *J. Infect. Dis.* **156**: 790.
186. Edman U, *et al.* (1990). *J. Exp. Med.* **172**: 879.
187. Arroyo R and Orozco E (1987). *Mol. Biochem. Parasitol.* **23**: 151.
188. García-Rivera G, *et al.* (1999). *Mol. Microbiol.* **33**: 556.
189. Bhattacharya A, *et al.* (1992). *Mol. Biochem. Parasitol.* **56**: 161.
190. Stanley Jr SL, *et al.* (1992). *Mol. Biochem. Parasitol.* **50**: 127.
191. Moody S, *et al.* (1997). *Parasitology* **114**: 95.
192. Moody S, *et al.* (1998). *J. Euk. Microbiol.* **45**: 9S.
193. Bhattacharya A, *et al.* (1999). *Parasitology* (In Press).
194. Martinets A, *et al.* (1997). *J. Exp. Med.* **186**: 1557.
195. Espinosa Cantellano M and Martínez-Palomo A (1991). *Biol. Cell* **72**: 189.
196. Avila EE and Calderón J (1993). *Exp. Parasitol.* **76**: 232.
197. Jacobs T, *et al.* (1998). *Mol. Microbiol.* **27**: 269.
198. Flores BM, *et al.* (1996). *J. Infect. Dis.* **173**: 226.
199. Zhang W-W and Samuelson J (1993). *Mol. Biochem. Parasitol.* **62**: 131.
200. Samuelson J, *et al.* (1990). *Mol. Biochem. Parasitol.* **38**: 281.
201. Descoteaux S, *et al.* (1992). *Mol. Biochem. Parasitol.* **54**: 201.

202. Shen P, *et al.* (1995). (Unpublished) GenBank Accession Number: U20321.
203. Martínez-Palomo A, *et al.* (1987) *Host-parasite cellular and molecular interactions in protozoal infections*, eds. Chang KP and Snary D (Springer-Verlag, Heidelberg) 371.
204. Serrano J de J, *et al.* (1996). *Parasitol. Res.* **82**: 200.
205. León G, *et al.* (1997). *Mol. Biochem. Parasitol.* **85**: 233.
206. Arhets P, *et al.* (1995). *Infect. Immun.* **63**: 4358.
207. Espinosa Cantellano M and Martínez-Palomo A (1994). *Exp. Parasitol.* **79**: 424.
208. Cox D, *et al.* (1995). *J. Cell Biol.* **128**: 819.
209. Tannich E (1999). (Unpublished) GenBank Accession Number: AF118397.
210. Talamás-Rohana P, *et al.* (1988). *J. Cell Biol.* **106**: 1787.
211. Talamás-Rohana P, *et al.* (1994). *Trans. R. Soc. Trop. Med. Hyg.* **88**: 596.
212. Talamás-Rohana P, *et al.* (1998). *J. Euk. Microbiol.* **45**: 356.
213. Mooseker MS and Cheney RE (1995). *Ann. Rev. Cell. Dev. Biol.* **11**: 633.
214. Jay PY, *et al.* (1995). *J. Cell Sci.* **108**: 387.
215. Soïd-Raggi LG, *et al.* (1998). *Exp. Parasitol.* **90**: 262.
216. Que X, *et al.* (1993). *Mol. Biochem. Parasitol.* **60**: 161.
217. Urban B, *et al.* (1996). *Mol. Biochem. Parasitol.* **80**: 171.
218. Samuelson J, *et al.* (1995). (Unpublished) GenBank Accession Numbers: U13418, U13419, U13420.
219. Guillén N, *et al.* (1998). *J. Cell Sci.* **111**: 1729.
220. Raha S, *et al.* (1994). *Mol. Biochem. Parasitol.* **65**: 63.
221. Muñoz M de L, *et al.* (1992). *Comp. Biochem. Physiol. [B]* **103**: 517.
222. Prasad J, *et al.* (1992). *Mol. Biochem. Parasitol.* **52**: 137.
223. Yadava N, *et al.* (1997). *Mol. Biochem. Parasitol.* **84**: 69.
224. Carbajal ME, *et al.* (1996). *Exp. Parasitol.* **82**: 11.
225. Manning-Cela R and Meza I (1997). *J. Euk. Microbiol.* **44**: 18.
226. Pérez E, *et al.* (1996). *Exp. Parasitol.* **82**: 164.
227. Santiago A, *et al.* (1994). *Exp. Parasitol.* **79**: 436.
228. Lioutas C, *et al.* (1995). *Exp. Parasitol.* **80**: 349.
229. Báez-Camargo M, *et al.* (1997). *Arch. Med. Res.* **28 (suppl.)**: S8. (Abstract)
230. Flores E, *et al.* (1997). *Arch. Med. Res.* **28 (suppl.)**: S5. (Abstract)
231. Bagchi A, *et al.* (1999). *Int. J. Parasitol.* (In Press).
232. Huang M, *et al.* (1997). *Arch. Med. Res.* **28 (suppl.)**: S1. (Abstract)
233. Cruz-Reyes J, *et al.* (1995). *Gene* **166**: 183.
234. Lohia A, *et al.* (1990). *Gene* **96**: 197.

235. Mittal V, *et al.* (1994). *Parasitology* **108**: 237.
236. Huber M, *et al.* (1989). *Mol. Biochem. Parasitol.* **32**: 285.
237. Bhattacharya S, *et al.* (1989). *J. Protozool.* **36**: 455.
238. Sehgal D, *et al.* (1994). *Mol. Biochem. Parasitol.* **67**: 205.
239. Bhattacharya S, *et al.* (1998). *Parasitol. Today* **14**: 181.
240. Bhattacharya S, *et al.* (1992). *Exp. Parasitol.* **74**: 200.
241. Sehgal D, *et al.* (1993). *Mol. Biochem. Parasitol.* **62**: 129.
242. Cázares F, *et al.* (1994). *Mol. Microbiol.* **12**: 607.
243. Dhar SK, *et al.* (1995). *Mol. Biochem. Parasitol.* **70**: 203.
244. Orozco E, *et al.* (1997). *Mol. Gen. Genet.* **254**: 250.
245. Báez Camargo M, *et al.* (1997). *Arch. Med. Res.* **28**: 5.
246. Albach RA (1989). *J. Protozool.* **36**: 197.
247. Luna-Arias JP, *et al.* (1999). *Microbiology* **145**: 33.
248. Urban B, *et al.* (1996). *Mol. Biochem. Parasitol.* **80**: 171.
249. Plaimauer B, *et al.* (1994). *Mol. Biochem. Parasitol.* **66**: 181.
250. Tannich E (1999). (Unpublished) GenBank Accession Number: AF11846.
251. Miranda R, *et al.* (1996).*Gene* **180**: 37.
252. Lioutas C and Tannich E (1995). *Mol. Biochem. Parasitol.* **73**: 259.
253. Shi XP, *et al.* (1997). *Biochim. Biophys. Acta* **1310**: 119.
254. De Meester F, *et al.* (1991). *Mol. Biochem. Parasitol.* **44**: 23.
255. Plaimauer B, *et al.* (1993). *DNA Cell Biol* **12**: 89.
256. Katiyar SK, *et al.* (1995). *Gene* **152**: 27.
257. Cevallos MA, *et al.* (1993). *Nucl. Acids Res.* **21**: 355.
258. Bhattacharya A (1997). (Unpublished) GenBank Accession Numbers: Y12250 and Y12251.
259. Bhattacharya A (1995). (Unpublished) GenBank Accession Number: X89635.
260. Novati S, *et al.* (1996). *Parasitology* **112**: 363.
261. Yamamoto A, *et al.* (1995). *Microbiol. Immunol.* **39**: 185.
262. Ramachandran S, *et al.* (1993). *Nucl. Acids Res.* **21**: 2011.
263. Eichinger DJ (1992). (Unpublished) GenBank Accession Number: Z11506.
264. Gangopadhyay SS, *et al.* (1997). *Mol. Biochem. Parasitol.* **89**: 73.
265. Makioka A, *et al.* (1997). *Parasitol. Int.* **46**: 27.
266. Makioka A, *et al.* (1998). *J. Parasitol.* **84**: 857.
267. Makioka A, *et al.* (1999). *Parasitol. Res.* **85**: 604.
268. Dhar SK, *et al.* (1996). *Mol. Cell Biol.* **16**: 2314.
269. Bhattacharya A, *et al.* (1999). *Curr. Sci.* **77**: 564
270. Blanc DS and Sargeaunt PG (1991). *Exp. Parasitol.* **72**: 87.

271. Jackson TFHG, *et al.* (1992). *Arch. Med. Res.* **23**: 71.
272. Jackson TFHG and Suparsad S (1997). *Arch. Med. Res.* **28 (suppl.)**: S304. (Abstract)
273. Diamond LS, *et al.* (1997). (Unpublished).
274. Sargeaunt PG (1987). *Parasitol. Today* **3**: 40.
275. Sargeaunt PG, *et al.* (1988). *Trans. R. Soc. Trop. Med. Hyg.* **82**: 862.
276. Gatti S, *et al.* (1997). *Parasitol. Res.* **83**: 716.
277. Clark CG and Diamond LS (1993). *Exp. Parasitol.* **77**: 450.
278. Samuelson J, *et al.* (1997). *Arch. Med. Res.* **28 (suppl.)**: S274. (Abstract)
279. Brumpt E (1928). *Trans. R. Soc. Trop. Med. Hyg.* **22**: 101.
280. Jackson TFHG and Ravdin JI (1996). *Parasitol. Today* **12**: 406.
281. Britten D, *et al.* (1997). *J. Clin. Microbiol.* **35**: 1108.
282. Mirelman D, *et al.* (1997). *J. Clin. Microbiol.* **35**: 2405.
283. Sanuki J, *et al.* (1996). *Parasitol. Res.* **83**: 96.
284. Haque R, *et al.* (1998). *J. Clin. Microbiol.* **36**: 449.
285. Coppi A and Eichinger D (1999). *Mol. Biochem. Parasitol.* **102**: 67.

Chapter 2

Epidemiology

Terry FHG Jackson

South African Medical Research Council
P. O. Box 17120, Congella 4013, South Africa
E-mail: jacksont@mrc.ac.za

Introduction

At the end of January 1997, a WHO/PAHO/UNESCO Expert Consultation was convened in Mexico City to evaluate the far reaching implications of recent developments in amebiasis. The work reviewed was initiated in the late 1970's (1), and incorporated biochemical, immunological and genetic studies of numerous scientists. In 1993, the accumulated data enabled a formal re-description of *E. histolytica*, the causative organism of amebiasis, to be tabled separating it from the morphologically identical *E. dispar* (2). Three publications (3–5) emanated from the WHO/PAHO/UNESCO consultation aimed at ensuring worldwide recognition of this re-description of *E. histolytica* in addition to disseminating the conclusions, recommendations and research needs identified by the consultants.

The realisation that *E. histolytica* and *E. dispar* are morphologically identical species with remarkably different physiological and pathological characteristics has impacted on all aspects of amebiasis but notably on the epidemiology. Furthermore, the weakness of our understanding of the epidemiology of amebiasis has been emphasised by these developments. Past epidemiological studies have erroneously always considered the two organisms together, albeit that *E. dispar* is a non-pathogenic intestinal commensal which occurs much more frequently in most populations than *E. histolytica*. On the other hand, *E. histolytica* is the causative organism of amebiasis. Consequently, the abovementioned Expert consultation recommended that the definition of amebiasis remains unchanged as, "infection with the protozoan parasite *E. histolytica*". In addition they identified weakness in our understanding of the epidemiology of amebiasis and four of the six research needs listed are epidemiologically based, namely:

- "Accurate prevalence data for *E. histolytica* are not available and obtaining them should be a high priority".
- "Molecular epidemiological studies should be vigorously pursued to determine whether some sub-groups of *E. histolytica* are more likely than others to cause invasive disease".
- "Data on the prevalence of asymptomatic carriers of *E. histolytica*, their likelihood of progressing to invasive disease, and the frequency of transmission to naive individuals are inadequate. More information in these areas is crucial for planning rational control strategies".
- "Knowledge of the host and parasite factors responsible for the invasiveness of *E. histolytica* is essential to understand how this organism causes disease".

In 1986, Walsh (6) assessed the existing global prevalence data and concluded that in 1981, 480 million people harboured *E. histolytica* worldwide. She went on to extrapolate that about 36 million develop clinically overt disease with 40–100,000 deaths each year, resulting in amebiasis ranking third, after malaria and schistosomiasis, as a parasitic cause of death. As this paper (6) attempted to estimate the global morbidity and mortality associated with amebiasis, it proved to be of great value to scientists working in this field and consequently it has been very widely quoted. As this paper appeared well before the formal re-description of *E. histolytica* was published (2), the epidemiological estimations quoted did not distinguish between *E. dispar* and *E. histolytica*. Revision of the prevalence and incidence estimations are necessary while that of mortality would remain the same. Unfortunately, reliable epidemiological data on populations that do not have selection bias and from whom confirmed *E. histolytica* and *E. dispar* isolations have been made, are rare. Such isolations from Durban, South Africa (7) have indicated the overall prevalence of both *E. histolytica* and *E. dispar* together to be 10%, with *E. histolytica* accounting proportionately for 1% and *E. dispar* for 9%. Interestingly, the situation in Durban may be a reflection of the overall estimates of 10% prevalence worldwide (6, 8, 9). Consequently, global prevalence of *E. histolytica* could be 50 million and that of *E. dispar*, 450 million.

Historical Background

A brief historical review follows in which the milestones in the discovery of *E. histoytica* and its host-parasite relationship are outlined to provide an insight into the research process that culminated in the re-description of *E. histolytica* (2).

Since the time of its first discovery in 1875 by Fedor Lösch (10), the causative organism of invasive amebiasis *E. histolytica* has been the centre of much controversy. Lösch described the presence of motile trophozoites in the dysenteric stools of a St Petersburg (Russia) labourer. He named the parasites 'Amoeba coli'. Lösch never attributed etiological significance to the presence of these amebas in the stool of the patient even though he not only successfully infected 4/5 dogs *per rectum* with them and demonstrated identical ulcerative lesions teeming with these so-called 'Amoeba coli' in both the dogs and the patient at autopsy. He attributed the dysentery to bacteria and concluded that the amebas merely served to perpetuate the inflammatory reaction.

Over the next 16 years many other authors confirmed Lösch's observation of concomitant infections with bacteria and amebas in dysenteric patients without making the association between the presence of amebas and dysentery. Reporting on their classic study in 1891, Councilman and Lafleur (11) (Baltimore) described the presence of 'Amoeba coli' in bacteriologically sterile liver abscess, thereby demonstrating the pathogenic potential of the organism independent of concomitant bacteria. They called the parasite 'Amoeba dysenteriae'.

The demonstration of cyst production by these pathogenic amebas enabled Quincke and Roos (12), two years later, to finally complete the picture of the life-cycle of 'Amoeba coli'; however they failed to adequately describe the specific characteristics of the cyst, such as the number of nuclei. Interestingly, they described successful infection of cats by both inoculation of trophozoites *per rectum* and feeding cysts *per os*. This is important as many authorities believe to this day that only primates can be successfully infected orally with cysts.

In 1897, asymptomatic healthy individuals were shown to asymptomatic-ally harbour a parasite named *Entamoeba coli* by Casagrandi and Barbagallo (13). The generic name *Entamoeba* was therefore established by these workers. Schaudinn (1903) (14) reserved the name *E. coli* for the non-pathogenic species and introduced the name *E. histolytica* for the dysentery producing ameba. Over the next few years, various authors recognised other *Entamoeba* species such as the quadrinucleate *E. tetragena* and the so-called small *E. minuta*.

This culminated in Kuenen and Swellengrebel (1913) (15), concluding that there were three forms in the life-cycle of *Entamoeba*: (i) the virulent histolytica stage in dysenteric stools, (ii) the avirulent stage in normal and convalescent subject's stools, and (iii) a cystic stage which was the progeny only of the avirulent forms which was responsible for propagation of the species. According to them, the histolytica phase, therefore, did not have any direct part to play in the life-cycle of the parasite.

The convoluted picture that had developed by this time could have been resolved by the risky, but nevertheless classical work, of Walker and Sellards (16), who in 1913, reported feeding cysts and trophozoites of *E. histolytica*, *E. coli* and free-living amebas from the Manila water supply to human volunteers. They proved conclusively that both free-living amebas and *E. coli* were non-pathogenic to humans. Of the 20 men fed with different strains of *E. coli*, 17 became parasitised and none developed any symptoms; they deduced that "*E. coli* is an obligatory parasite… and that it is non-pathogenic and consequently plays no role in the etiology of entamoebic dysentery". Furthermore they stated that *E. tetragena* was identical to *E. histolytica* and that *E. minuta* was the pre-encysted stage of *E. histolytica*. However, of all their feeding experiments, the most definitive ever conducted on this topic was accomplished by feeding cysts obtained from a carrier convalescing from amebic dysentery, to three volunteers. This resulted in 2 of them developing amebic dysentery while the third proved to be an asymptomatic cyst passer. Cysts obtained from one of the dysenteric subjects colonised but failed to produce dysentery in a further 3 volunteers. Two other volunteers fed with cysts from the asymptomatic carrier became asymptomatically parasitised, and when cysts from one of these subjects were in turn fed to 4 other persons, dysentery developed in one, 2 others were asymptomatically colonised, while the fourth was not successfully colonised. This study proved that *E. histolytica* can give rise to both invasive amebiasis and asymptomatic infection; furthermore, cysts from asymptomatically infected subjects can cause invasive amebiasis. Although this study provided the key to understanding *Entamoeba* spp, insufficient attention was paid to the work and 70–80 contentious years followed before modern biochemical methods were used to reconfirm these findings!

By 1917, it was widely accepted that the quadrinucleate cysts of the tetragena type were those of *E. histolytica*. It became increasingly apparent that there was a gross discrepancy between the prevalence of the parasite and active disease; furthermore it was not possible to predict the appearance of dysentery in asymptomatic individuals. In attempting to explain the poor correlation between the prevalence of cyst passers and that of invasive disease, three broad schools of thought developed:

(1) *Promethean Theory* (17) — Based on the mythical Greek character Prometheus who had his tissues devoured all day by an eagle after nocturnal regeneration to compensate for the ravages of the previous day. *E. histolytica* was perceived to be an obligatory tissue parasite which normally survived in equilibrium with its host, causing development of disease in its host only when there was a loss in the host's ability to tolerate the parasite. Major concerns with this theory were raised when it was realised that the parasites in *in vitro* culture could happily survive on bacteria in the absence of human tissues.

(2) *Commensal Theory* (15) — *E. histolytica* was viewed as a gut commensal which was responsible for propagation of the species. Some as yet unconfirmed stimulus (e.g. nature of gut flora, dietary implications, rapid passage) caused the ameba to mutate into a tissue invading form which lost its capability of cyst production and therefore effectively committed suicide as transmission to another host was impossible. This concept was popular with scientists right up to recent times even though the hypothetical trigger responsible for the mutation escaped acceptable scientific resolution.

(3) *Two Species Theory* (18) — Brumpt in 1928, noting the difference in prevalence of invasive amebiasis in tropical climates and temperate areas, put forward the concept that *E. histolytica* comprised two morphologically identical species. The one, which he named *E. dispar*, was proposed to be non-pathogenic and confined to temperate zones, where in spite of a relatively high prevalence of asymptomatic carriers, the prevalence of disease was low. The other, *E. dysenteriae*, he postulated was the pathogenic species (as its name implies) responsible for invasive amebiasis; in addition he claimed that this species was more prevalent in tropical zones where the prevalence of disease was considerably higher. In his opinion, it was possible to have healthy carriers of *E. dysenteriae* in whom there was mild tissue invasion, the amebas in such cases feeding predominantly on bacteria; if for some reason the host's defences were compromised, *E. dysenteriae* invaded the deeper tissues giving rise to symptoms. Such changes in the host defence mechanisms however, did not have any effect on the invasive capability of *E. dispar*. Both *E. dispar* and *E. dysenteriae* had independent life-cycles, both of them producing quadrinucleate cysts which were morphologically identical.

Although Brumpt's hypothesis best described the epidemiology of the parasite and has proved to be closest to current beliefs based on modern scientific analysis of the organism, it was never widely accepted during the following 50 years.

Sargeaunt (1) working from the London School of Hygiene and Tropical Medicine introduced isoenzyme electrophoresis to study polymorphism in the intestinal protozoa of man. Between 1978 and 1987, he worked with scientists from Mexico, India, Japan, Australia, Israel and, most extensively, South Africa (19). The outcome after studying approximately 10,000 amebic isolates was the realisation that Brumpt had been correct and that ther were indeed two morphologically identical species that had up to this stage been grouped together as one organism, *E. histolytica*. As early as 1982 (20) he suggested that we revert to the nomenclature proposed by Emile Brumpt — *E. dispar* and *E. dysenteriae*.

In 1986, Mirelman's group from the Weizman Institute in Israel published results of experimental conversion from one species to the other, apparently induced by changing culture conditions (21). This work could not be reliably reproduced by their group on all the isolates they studied. Furthermore, other independent laboratories with considerable experience in the field, reported from various parts of the world that they could not reproduce the work. These observed conversions are now considered by most to either be culture contamination or artifacts of the highly artificial culture environment in which they apparently occurred.

Shortly after this Tannich of Bernhard Nocht Institute in Hamburg, Germany elegantly confirmed the observations of Sargeaunt by means of DNA studies (22). In 1991, Clark and Diamond of NIH went on to reconfirm Tannich's observations using ribo-printing; they also pointed out that the estimated genetic distance between the two species was as great as that between man and mouse (23). As mentioned in the introduction, they subsequently proposed that these two species be named *E. dispar* and *E. histolytica* (2). The latter is the causative organism of invasive amebiasis. The former is widely believed to be a gut commensal. This nomenclature is now in usage worldwide.

The Strains of *E. histolytica* and *E. dispar*

As early as 1968, Reeves and Bischoff (24) employed isoenzyme electrophoresis for the preliminary characterisation of *Entamoeba*. Ten years later, Sargeaunt *et al.* (1) initiated an in-depth series of studies, based on isoenzyme electrophoresis in starch gel, to characterise the intestinal amebas of man. However they focussed on E. histolytica and E. dispar. Robinson's medium (25) was preferred as a means of primary isolation as it favours the growth of these two amebas. The isoenzyme systems chosen were malic enzyme (ME), phosphoglucomutase (PGM), glucose phosphate isomerase (GPI) and hexokinase (HK). As ME migrates to the same position from the origin for both E. histolytica and E. dispar it is used to confirm their presence. The migration band closest to the origin can be used to differentiate between them, as the band migrates further in both cases in the presence of E. histolytica. By examining the characteristic banding patterns of PGM and GPI simultaneously it is possible to place the amebas into one of more than 20 zymodemes (strains allocated on the basis of the particular isoenzyme patterns observed). All these zymodemes were attributed to E. histolytica before its separation from E. dispar was accepted, but most importantly, they were categorised as pathogenic zymodemes (PZ) and non-pathogenic zymodemes (NPZ), according to their observed association with invasive amebiasis. Consequently PZ is a synonym for E. histolytica and NPZ for E. dispar.

Of the 20 zymodemes that Sargeaunt (26) isolated, 9 proved to be those of E. histolytica (PZ) while the rest were E. dispar (NPZ). Isoenzymes have been widely employed as tools to monitor genetic differences both intra- and inter-specifically. However, the value of isoenzyme differentiation in the case of E. histolytica has been controversial. A pivotal event in the controversy resulted from the reported observation (21) that E. histolytica could be converted into E. dispar and vice versa by varing the culture conditions in which it was maintained. This phenomenon was refuted after several years when established laboratories reported that they could not reproduce the work and Clark et al. (27) formally declared these isoenzyme conversions to be artifactual. Isoenzymes (PGM and HK in particular) can therefore be reliably used to distinguish between the two species of ameba, E. histolytica and E. dispar.

As mentioned above, the zymodeme is determined by examining the patterns of PGM and GPI; these have either single or multiple banding patterns. The zymodemes were numbered chronologically. Typically therefore in a survey in which the zymodemes are determined it will be found that those with the lowest numbers (I, II, III) are encountered most frequently. The exception is zymodeme XIV (E. histolytica) which is prevalent in India and was described chronologically later after Sargeaunt commenced his surveys in India (28). Zymodeme XIV is by far the most prevalent zymodeme of E. histolytica in India although zymodeme II has been reported (29).

Interestingly, in surveys in South Africa shifts between the single and double banded zymodemes of both *E. dispar* and *E. histolytica* (30) have been observed; furthermore, zymodeme XI (*E. histolytica*- multiple banded) has been isolated from the gut while zymodeme II (*E. histolytica*- single banded) was isolated from the liver abscess of the same patient and *vice versa* (31). This led to the proposal that the single banded zymodemes (I — *E. dispar*; II and XIV — *E. histoytica*) reflect the genotype of the parasite while the multiple banded zymodemes are phenotypic (30–32). Upon axenising zymodemes I, II, III, XI and XIV Jackson *et al.* (32) found that the pattern of the single banded zymodemes (I, II and XIV) remained unchanged while the multiple banded zymodemes reverted to the most appropriate single banded one (III to I; XI to II). It is therefore likely that the true genotypic strains are far more limited in number than the range of zymodemes indicated initially. Determination of the exact zymodeme in epidemiological surveys is therefore of limited value, while the differentiation of *E. histolytica* from *E. dispar* by isoenzyme electrophoresis is invaluable.

Interestingly, the reversion of multiple banded zymodemes to single banded zymodemes has proved to be a consistent feature except in the case of zymodeme XIX (33). Zymodeme XIX has been isolated most commonly from persons who acquired their infections in Africa but it has also originated from India, Burma and Thailand (34, 35). It has an unusual triple banding pattern in GPI where subdivision of the band furtherest from the origin appears to have occurred. When this zymodeme was axenised, it retained its banding pattern (33). If this phenomenon implies that zymodeme XIX is a genotypic strain of *E. histolytica*, it seems that 3 strains (II, XIV and XIX) of *E. histolytica* can be identified by isoenzyme electrophoresis. Two of them (XIV — India; XIX — usually Africa) apparently originate from certain geographical regions, while the third (II) has a worldwide distribution.

Studies conducted at the DNA level have been invaluable for differentiating between *E. histolytica* and *E. dispar*. Clark and Diamond (36) recently described a technique known as "riboprinting" which permits differentiation by examination of restriction enzyme site polymorphisms in PCR-amplified small subunit ribosomal RNA genes. It seems that riboprinting can be used for both intra- and inter-specific differentiation. Molecular epidemiological tools such as this should be valuable in future for establishing infection pathways as they will enable genetic fingerprinting of intra-specific strains in addition to differentiating between *E. histolytica* and *E. dispar*.

Parasite and Disease Distribution

Although the definition of amebiasis is "infection with the protozoan parasite *E. histolytica*" the distribution of both this parasite and *E. dispar* will be considered in this section as they have been considered together in past epidemiological texts.

Information on the geographical distribution of the parasite and amebiasis is incomplete and unreliable. Surveys have not been conducted using standard procedures and in only a few differentiation of *E. histolytica* and *E. dispar* has been attempted. Elsdon-Dew (36) was requested by the WHO to review available literature on parasite prevalence but he concluded that little reliance could be placed on the majority of the data. However, using his findings and those of Walsh (6), certain generalisations can be made. Firstly, *E. histolytica* and *E. dispar* have a worldwide distribution, being found in cold, temperate, and tropical climates. In the past they did not seem to occur in Eskimos and Poles (90,000 examinations) (37, 38). They are both more prevalent in disadvantaged communities and in tropical areas. This is believed to be related to poorer sanitation, nutrition and decreased resistance in those living in these environments. Recognized high-risk areas for acquiring amebiasis, include Mexico, the western portion of South America, West Africa, South Africa (particularly in the black population), parts of the Middle East, and South and Southeast Asia. Invasive disease seems to be more common in these areas. Many of the cases identified in North America and in Europe are imported, but a level of endemicity is present and occasional water-borne epidemics have occurred.

Seasonal variations in prevalence of the parasite have been recorded. Usually the onset of the rainy season is associated with a sharp rise in prevalence (39, 40), followed by a fall as the rains progress (40). However, high prevalence of infection has been reported in Nigeria during the dry months of the year, associated with the use of contaminated water resulting from limited supplies (41). In addition to temperature and rainfall, humidity also seems to be a contributing factor in parasite transmission with records of markedly higher prevalence at the coast (52.3%) when compared to the highlands (13.7%) (40).

Accurate determination of the true prevalence of amebiasis is difficult. Surveyed populations may differ, and the prevalence in certain groups is higher than in the general population, e.g. in families of infected patients, in male homosexuals, and in persons in mental hospitals, prisons, and institutions for children. Differences in laboratory techniques, competence of laboratory personnel, stool collection methods, intermittent excretion of cysts in the stool and number of specimens examined from each person may lead to either under- or over-diagnosis. Most studies rely on examination of one stool specimen. This approach will detect only 40–50% of those infected while three consecutive examinations on separate days can be expected to yield 60–80%; > 90% can be identified if more than five examinations are performed (6). A study in the Gambia using single stool examinations indicated that an average of 20–30% of the population excreted cysts at any one time, but longitudinal follow-up over a year proved that almost all the study subjects (> 98%) excreted cysts at some time (40).

Sexual transmission of *Entamoeba* has been widely documented, especially amongst homosexual men (42–44). In 1978, the New York City Department of Health recorded 1875 infections with *E. histolytica/E. dispar* in the male homosexual population; this exceeded city totals for most of the other major infectious diseases of public health importance, such as tuberculosis (1307) and hepatitis (1260), and approached that of primary and secondary syphilis (2060) (42). In Toronto, Canada *E. histolytica/E. dispar* infections were observed in 27% of homosexual men compared to only 1% of heterosexual men (43) and notably no cases of amebic colitis or liver abscess were documented in any of these cases. In London, isoenzyme electrophoretic studies revealed that 11.1% of male homosexuals harboured *E. dispar* (44). These three reports are a few of the substantial number in which it appears that homosexuals in western countries have a high prevalence of infection with non-pathogenic *E. dispar* based most commonly on the absence of clinical symptoms and negative serology as well as a few reports employing isoenzyme characterisation. It is however highly unlikely that male homosexuals in western countries are refractory to infection with pathogenic *E. histolytica*. This is borne out by a case of amebic liver abscess in a male homosexual described by Thompson *et al.* (45) and by reports from Japan where amebic infection was first observed in male homosexuals with invasive amebiasis and where more than 50 cases have been detected (46). The anomaly observed in western countries could be explained in part by the large reservoir of the more commonly occurring *E. dispar*, maintained in the male homosexual population, and as an outcome of many studies recruiting study subjects from Sexually Transmitted Disease clinics in preference to Gastroenterology clinics. Considering the comments in the previous paragraph it is likely that the incidence rates in most male homosexual populations would be about 100% over a one year period.

In a study of 1381 asymptomatic individuals living in a semirural endemic area south of Durban, South Africa *E. dispar* occurred more frequently in females of all age groups whereas *E. histolytica* was equally common in males and females (7). In a subsequent longitudinal study of asymptomatic carriers of *E. histolytica*, infections with this organism were equally common in males and females (30). This is at variance with the higher prevalence of invasive amebiasis in males than females, which has been reported to be in a ratio of 2 : 1 (males : females) in patients with amebic dysentery and 7 : 1 in patients with amebic liver abscess (47). It seems that while males and females have an equal chance of being asymptomatically infected with *E. histolytica*, females are protected by some mechanism from acquiring invasive amebiasis. It is noteworthy that in this study (30) the prevalence of asymptomatic *E. histolytica* infection in the 5–15 year age group, in which invasive amebiasis is believed to be extremely rare (47), was similar to that in the > 16 year age group, in which invasive amebiasis is most commonly diagnosed (47). Why certain age groups and females should be refractory to invasion by the parasite is unknown and needs further study.

In a semi-rural area south of Durban, South Africa 9% of asymptomatic individuals were found to be infected with non-pathogenic *E. dispar* while 1% were infected with *E. histolytica* (7). The 1% with *E. histolytica* represent a public health hazard as they are reservoirs of infection with a pathogenic organism. Asymptomatic carriers are more likely to spread the disease than symptomatic patients with invasive amebiasis as the latter individuals will seek medical attention. The necessity to identify and treat asymptomatic carriers of *E. histolytica* is emphasised by the observation that 10% of them develop invasive amebiasis in due course (30). In those that do not develop invasive amebiasis "self-cure" apparently occurs within 12 months (30); this observation concurs with that of Nanda *et al.* (48) who followed subjects in India with both *E. histolytica* and *E. dispar* and found that all had apparently undergone "self-cure" within 19 months. It is important to note that the serological response in asymptomatic carriers of *E. histolytica* is as marked as that seen in patients with invasive amebiasis, implying sub-clinical tissue invasion (48).

E. histolytica occurs more frequently in family groups and closely associated individuals (30). This phenomenon has been reported by others (49, 50) in studies in which differentiation between *E. histolytica* and *E. dispar* was not attempted, and highlights the importance of direct person to person transmission. Overcrowding can therefore be expected to increase incidence rates. Furthermore, the persistence of infection with *E. histolytica* for 6–12 months without developing invasive amebiasis provides good evidence that a carrier state does exist. Good public health practice would require follow-up and treatment where necessary of all contacts of patients with invasive amebiasis as well as asymptomatic carriers of *E. histolytica*.

Epidemiological Indices

A number of indices have been used to assess the incidence and prevalence of invasive amebiasis and the distribution of the parasites associated with this disease. Each has advantages and disadvantages. The formal re-description of *E. histolytica* and *E. dispar* (2) as separate species and the development of refined tools for identifying them has widened the range of available epidemiological indices. More meaningful epidemiological surveys can now be conducted and hopefully in future years data will be gathered that will obviate the lament of Elsdon-Dew (36) who on summing up an epidemiological review he had written stated, "the only value of this report is to show that it has none". These indices are discussed below:

Frequency of invasive amebiasis

Owing to the widespread practice of regarding dysentery of unknown origin as amebic (36), the frequency of intestinal amebiasis is not a useful index of invasive amebiasis. Few reports of intestinal amebiasis include the essential microscopic observations of *E. histolytica* trophozoites and sigmoidoscopic investigation for ulcerative lesions (51). A further restriction is that intestinal amebiasis is seen in disproportionally low numbers compared to hepatic amebiasis in hospitals in endemic areas probably as a result of rapid and effective treatment by medical practitioners and clinics.

The frequency of hepatic amebiasis is a reliable measure of morbidity as the lesion can be identified relatively easily, in the laboratory or by postmortem studies. As hepatic amebiasis is not normally a notifiable disease, the majority of cases are not reported in public health statistics. Its value as an index of invasive amebiasis is therefore limited to specific local studies.

Stool microscopy and serology

These two indices are usually considered separately. Since it is possible to use them together to enhance the outcome of epidemiological surveys, they are dealt with in combination in this section.

As a result of the re-description of *E. histolytica* and *E. dispar* (2) reliance on microscopy alone for their detection is no longer appropriate as their cysts are morphologically identical. A further restriction is that microscopy is relatively insensitive when performed on a single specimen (40–50%) (6), with culture yielding up to a four-fold increase in sensitivity for parasite detection (7); however > 90% of cyst passers can be identified if more than 5 consecutive specimens are examined (6). In addition it must be remembered that up to 90% of human infections reported in the past to be *E. histolytica*, were in fact, intestinal colonisation with the morphologically identical *E. dispar* (7). This highlights the poor specificity of microscopy when used on its own.

Currently available serologic tests usually employ antigen prepared from axenically cultured *E. histolytica*. When these are used in conjunction with isoenzyme characterisation of isolated amebas, *E. histolytica* and not *E. dispar* is responsible for eliciting a serological response in humans whether they are symptomatic or not (48, 52). Consequently, this enables a useful, relatively rapid method, using a combination of serology and microscopy, for differentiating between *E. histolytica* and *E. dispar*. Regardless of symptoms, the presence of quadrinucleate cysts in the stool and a negative serologic response indicates that the cysts are those of *E. dispar*. Furthermore, in an endemic area a positive serologic response indicates current or remote infection with *E. histolytica*, and in non-endemic regions, sero-positivity has a high diagnostic specificity for current *E. histolytica* infection (52, 53).

The major advantage of combining stool microscopy and serology is that data can be gathered at any site where these two widely used techniques are employed.

Isoenzyme electrophoresis

As an index, isoenzyme electrophoresis of amebas isolated by culture (1) is currently the gold standard for epidemiological studies as *E. histolytica* and *E. dispar* can be reliably differentiated. This method has played a key role in enhancing our understanding of amebiasis and in determining that the causative organism is a member of a newly redescribed species complex (2). It is a time consuming and fastidious process and as a result has been limited to a few laboratories in various parts of the world. More streamlined methods are replacing isoenzyme electrophoresis and these will be discussed briefly below.

Antigen capture tests

The development of assays for detection of amebic antigen in faeces has been designated a priority in amebiasis research by the WHO (54). Antigen capture assays offer many advantages over existing tests such as identification of the currency of infection, indication of extent of infection, increased objectivity and the potential for automation. Numerous groups have described antigen capture ELISA's that could not differentiate between *E. histolytica* and *E. dispar* (55). Two groups have described ELISA's that can differentiate between these two species of amebas (56, 57) and a third group (58) has developed an ELISA that is specific for *E. histolytica* thereby allowing identification of infections with *E. dispar* to be made by deduction. The ELISA of Abd-Alla (57) has successfully detected antigen in both serum and stool thereby enhancing its value. As they are relatively rapid, sensitive and specific these very promising antigen capture tests are expected to become more widely used as epidemiological indices.

Nucleic acid studies

Undoubtedly, the epidemiological indices of the future will be based on nucleic acid detection methods such as the polymerase chain reaction (PCR). As these techniques offer high specificity and sensitivity, are capable of detecting minute amounts of parasite material and are fast, they have the potential to be the indices of choice in the future. Recent reports such as those of Acuna-Soto *et al.* (59) and Rivera *et al.* (60) confirm the potential value of PCR in field studies. Clark and Diamond (36) described a technique known as "riboprinting" which permits differentiation by examination of restriction enzyme site polymorphisms in PCR-amplified small subunit ribosomal RNA genes. Apparently riboprinting can be used for both intra- and inter-specific differentiation. Indices such as this should be valuable in future for establishing infection pathways as they will enable genetic fingerprinting of intra-specific strains in addition to differentiating between *E. histolytica* and *E. dispar*.

References

1. Sargeaunt PG, Williams JE and Grene JD (1978). *Trans. R. Soc. Trop. Med. Hyg.* **72**: 519–521.
2. Diamond LS and Clark CG (1993). *J. Euk. Microbiol.* **40**: 340–344.

3. World Health Organisation (1997). *Weekly Epidemiol. Rec.* **72**: 97–99.
4. Pan American Health Organisation (1997). *Epidemiol. Bull.* **18**: 13–14.
5. World Health Organisation (1997). *Bull. WHO* **75**: 291–292.
6. Walsh JA (1986). *Rev. Infect. Dis.* **8**: 228–238.
7. Gathiram V and Jackson TFHG (1985). *Lancet* **i**: 719–721.
8. Martinez-Palomo A (1986). *Clinics in Tropical Medicine and Communicable Diseases*, ed. Gilles HM (Saunders, London) 587–601.
9. Reed SL (1992). *Clin Infect. Dis.* **14**: 385–393.
10. Losch FD (1875). *Anatomie und Physiologie* **65**: 196–211.
11. Councilman WT and Lafleur HA (1891). *Johns Hopkins Hosp. Bull.* **2**: 395–548.
12. Quinke H and Roos E (1893). *Berl. klin Wschr.* **30**: 1089–1094.
13. Casagrandi O and Barbagallo P (1897). *Ann. Igiene* **7**: 103–117.
14. Schaudinn F (1903). *Arbeit. Kaiserlichen Gesundheitsamte* **19**: 547–576.
15. Kuenen WA and Swellengrebel NH (1913). *Centralblatt fur Bakteriologie* **71**: 378–410.
16. Walker EL and Sellards AW (1913). Experimental entamoebic dysentery. *Phillipine Journal of Science* **8B**: 253–331.
17. Dobell C (1918). *J. Trop. Med. Hyg.* **21**: 115–119.
18. Brumpt E (1928). *Trans. Roy. Soc. Trop. Med. Hyg.* **22**: 101–124.
19. Sargeaunt PG (1987). *Parasitol. Today* **3**: 40–43.
20. Sargeaunt PG, *et al.* (1982). *Arch. Med. Res.* **13**: 89–94.
21. Mirelman D, *et al.* (1986). *Exp. Parasitol.* **62**: 142–148.
22. Tannich E, Horstmann RD, Knobloch J and Arnold HH (1989). *Proc. Natl. Acad. Sci., U.S.A.* **86**: 5118–5122.
23. Clark CG and Diamond LS (1991). *Mol. Biochem. Parasitol.* **49**: 297–302.
24. Reeves RE and Bischoff JM (1968). *J. Parasitol.* **54**: 594–600.
25. Robinson GL (1968). *Trans. Roy. Soc. Trop. Med. Hyg.* **62**: 285–294.
26. Sargeaunt PG (1988). *Amebiasis. Human Infection by Entamoeba histolytica*, ed. Ravdin J (John Wiley & Sons, New York) 370–387.
27. Clark CG, Cunnick CC and Diamond LS (1992). *Exp. Parasitol.* **74**: 307–314.
28. Sargeaunt PG, Baveja UK, Nanda R and Anand BS (1984). *Trans. Roy. Soc. Trop. Med. Hyg.* **78**: 96–101.
29. Baveja UK, Francis S, Kaur M and Agarwal SK (1990). *J. Diarrhoeal Dis. Res.* **8**: 27–30.
30. Gathiram V and Jackson TFHG (1987). *S. Afr. Med. J.* **72**: 669–672.

31. Irusen EM, Jackson TFHG and Simjee AE (1992). *Clin. Infect. Dis.* **14**: 889–893.
32. Jackson TFHG, Gathiram V, Suparsad S and Anderson CB (1992). *Arch. Med. Res.* **23**: 71.
33. Jackson TFHG and Suparsad S (1997). *Arch. Med. Res.* **28**: 304–305.
34. Sargeaunt PG (1985). *Trans. Roy. Soc. Trop. Med. Hyg.* **79**: 86–89.
35. Sargeaunt PG, Jackson TFHG, Wiffen SR and Bhojnani R (1988). *Trans. Roy. Soc. Trop. Med. Hyg.* **82**: 862–867.
36. Elsdon-Dew R (1968). *Adv. Parasitol.* **6**: 1–62.
37. Brown M, Green JE, Boag TJ and Kuitenen-Ekbaum E (1954). *Can. J. Publ. Hlth.* **3**: 508.
38. Laird M and Meerovitch E (1961). *Can. J. Zool.* **39**: 63–67.
39. Nzeako BC (1992). *J. Commun. Dis.* **24**: 224–230.
40. Bray RS and Harris WG (1977). *Trans. Roy. Soc. Trop. Med. Hyg.* **71**: 401–407.
41. Ogunba EO (1977). *J. Trop. Med. Hyg.* **80**: 187–191.
42. Pommerantz BM, Marr JS and Goldman WD (1980). *Bull. N. Y. Acad. Med.* **56**: 232–244.
43. Keystone JS, Keystone DL and Proctor EM (1980). *Can. Med. Assoc. J.* **123**: 512–514.
44. Sargeaunt PG, *et al.* (1983). *Br. J. Vener. Dis.* **59**: 193–195.
45. Thompson JE, Freischlag J and Thomas DS (1983). *Sex. Transm. Dis.* **10**: 153–155.
46. Takeuchi T, *et al.* (1990). *Trans. Roy. Soc. Trop. Med. Hyg.* **84**: 250–251.
47. Wilmot AJ (1973). *Clinical Medicine in Africans in Southern Africa*, eds. Campbell GD, Seedat YK and Daynes G (Churchill-Livingstone, Edinburgh) 3–15.
48. Jackson TFHG, Gathiram V and Simjee AE (1985). *Lancet* i: 716–718.
49. Dykes AC, *et al.* (1980). *Pediatrics* **65**: 799–803.
50. Spencer HC, *et al.* (1977). *Am. J. Trop. Med. Hyg.* **26**: 628–635.
51. Munoz O (1986). *Amebiasis*, ed. Martinez-Palomo A (Elsevier Science Publishers, BV) 213–239.
52. Ravdin JI, *et al.* (1990). *J. Infect. Dis.* **162**: 768–772.
53. Abd-Alla M, El-Hawey AM and Ravdin JI (1992). *Am. J. Trop. Med. Hyg.* **47**: 800–804.
54. World Health Organisation (1991). *WHO/PAHO Informal Consultation on Intestinal Protozoal Infections* (Oaxtepec, Mexico) 5–10.
55. Jackson TFHG and Ravdin JI (1996). *Parasitol. Today* **12**: 406–409.

56. Haque R, *et al.* (1993). *J. Infect. Dis.* **167**: 247–249.
57. Abd-Alla M, *et al.* (1993). *J. Clin. Microbiol.* **31**: 2845–2850.
58. Gonzales-Ruiz A, *et al.* (1994). *J. Clin. Microbiol.* **32**: 964–970.
59. Acuno-Soto R, *et al.* (1993). *Am. J. Trop. Med. Hyg.* **48**: 58–70.
60. Rivera WL, *et al.* (1996). *Parasitol. Res.* **82**: 585–589.

Chapter 3

Mechanisms of Host Resistance

D Campbell and K Chadee

Department of Parasitology of McGill University
Macdonald Campus, 21,111 Lakeshore Rd.
Ste. Anne de Bellevue, Quebec, H9X 3V9, Canada
E-mail: kris_chadee@maclan.mcgill.ca

Tissue invasion by *E. histolytica* stimulates cell-mediated and humoral immune responses. Although innate defences may retard amebic invasion, acquired immunity is required for host defence and resistance to reinfection. Antigen-specific T cells directly lyse amebas *in vitro* and produce cytokines such as Interferon-γ that activate macrophages for *in vitro* amebicidal activity. Killing of *E. histolytica* by activated macrophages appears to be a major mechanism involved in anti-amebic defence. Depletion of macrophages *in vivo* allows or exacerbates amebic liver abscess development. *In vitro*, macrophages activated by recombinant cytokines exhibit potent amebic killing by a nitric oxide-dependent mechanism. Activated neutrophils and eosinophils express *in vitro* amebicidal activity and possibly contribute to control of infection *in vivo*. Antibody production does not correlate with protection against *E. histolytica*; ameba can cap and ingest or proteolytically degrade antibodies attached to its surface. In a primary invasive infection, acute disease is associated with suppression of cell-mediated immunity (CMI). In contrast, drug-cured patients and animals as well as immunized animals, which are resistant to challenge infection, displayed potent CMI responses *in vitro*. Hence, development of effective CMI appears key in controlling or resisting invasive amebiasis.

Introduction

Intestinal and extra-intestinal disease caused by *E. histolytica* occurs worldwide with a preponderance of cases reported in developing countries.

Approximately 40 million people suffer from amebic colitis or amebic liver abscess (ALA) annually, and between 40,000 and 110,000 of these individuals die of the disease (1). However, patients who recover from amebiasis may acquire some level of resistance to reinfection. A recurrence rate of only 0.29% was reported in a 5-year study of ALA patients in Mexico (2), a level much lower than would have been expected in an endemic area. In addition, intestinal colonization by amebas appeared to be a less frequent event for seropositive individuals (evidence of past exposure to infection) than for those who were seronegative (3). Using animal models of the disease, it has been repeatedly demonstrated that various immunization regimes with defined amebic antigens generate protective immunity (4). Cumulatively, human and animal studies indicate that resistance to reinfection with *E. histolytica* may occur.

Due to the paucity of reagents for immunological studies in the gerbil (principal animal model of hepatic amebiasis (5)) and the lack of a immuno-competent murine model, detailed analysis of the immune basis for resistance to *E. histolytica* has lagged behind the analysis of immunological resistance to other major parasitic diseases such as leishmaniasis and malaria. Both humoral and cell-mediated immune responses to *E. histolytica* develop in natural human infections and in experimentally-induced animal infections. However, amebas have multiple immunomodulatory effects on host responses. T cell and macrophage-mediated defense as well as anti-amebic effects of antibodies can be countered by the parasite. Recent advancements such as the description of ALA formation in severe combined immunodeficient (SCID) mice (6) and the development of new reagents for immunological studies in gerbils (7) are helping to elucidate mechanisms of resistance to *E. histolytica*. In this chapter, we shall examine current proposed mechanisms of resistance to *E. histolytica* supported by *in vitro* and *in vivo* studies.

Innate Resistance Mechanisms

Initial host resistance to *E. histolytica* is dependent on natural or innate resistance mechanisms prior to the development of acquired immunity. Amebas encounter natural "barriers" to infection in both the gut and systemic circulation following tissue invasion. These innate defences may prevent or partially inhibit amebic tissue invasion, although the level of protection afforded by innate resistance is difficult to quantify precisely. Mucins lining the colonic epithelium provide an important innate defence against tissue invasion by *E. histolytica*. Amebas bound rat and human colonic mucins with high affinity via the 170 kDa heavy subunit of the parasite's Gal/GalNAc adherence lectin (Gal-lectin) (8). This binding inhibited amebic adherence to and cytolysis of target cells. Therefore, mucins serve as a first line of host defence in the gut by inhibiting amebic attachment to the underlying mucosal epithelial cells. It is hypothesized that amebic-derived mucin secretagogues promote depletion of mucins, enabling amebas to attach to and lyse colonic epithelial cells (9). In the gut, other factors such as competition by intestinal bacteria for attachment to mucins may inhibit amebic colonization (10).

In the systemic circulation, *E. histolytica* is exposed to complement, another innate resistance mechanism that may act to decrease the numbers of invading amebas. Amebas activated both the alternative and classical complement pathways in normal serum (i.e. in the absence of anti- amebic antibodies) (11). Hamsters depleted of complement by treatment with cobra venom factor suffered increased susceptibility to ALA formation (12), demonstrating the *in vivo* relevance of complement-mediated killing. However, amebas have been shown to develop complement resistance after successive exposure to with human serum (13). While both complement resistant and susceptible amebas activated complement, only the latter were killed (14). These results suggest that complement resistance is necessary for tissue invasion. The Gal-lectin molecule has sequence homology and antigenic cross-reactivity with CD59, a membrane inhibitor of C5b-9 in human erythrocytes, suggesting the Gal-lectin also has complement-inhibitory functions (15). Experiments demonstrated that the Gal-lectin bound C8 and C9, effectively preventing assembly of the C5b-C9 membrane attack complex and subsequent cell lysis (15). A specific role for the Gal-lectin was confirmed by abrogation of amebic complement resistance following treatment with a monoclonal antibody (mAb) to the Gal-lectin (15).

Acquired Resistance Mechanisms

Tissue invasion by *E. histolytica* trophoziotes results in the rapid development of acquired immune responses that may limit the primary infection and/or provide the sensitized host with protection against repeat infections. Amebas are able to sustain themselves in host tissues possibly through modulation of the immune response to the parasite. Prior sensitization through immunization or previous parasite exposure may enable the immune system to destroy trophoziotes before they manipulate the host response. Evidence from *in vivo* and *in vitro* studies suggests that protective immunity primarily involves cell-mediated responses, however humoral responses may also contribute to anti-amebic defence.

T Cell Responses

A role for antigen-specific T cells in controlling invasive amebiasis is evident from studies demonstrating that thymectomy or treatment with anti-T lymphocyte serum resulted in exacerbation of infection in animal models of the disease (16–18). Additionally, in athymic nude (nu/nu) Balb/c mice, which lack functional T cells, amebic caecal infections were prolonged (19). Conversely, it has been demonstrated that passive transfer of immunity against hepatic amebiasis in hamsters using spleen cells was dependent on T cells (20).

T cells respond to amebic infections or immunization with amebic molecules by proliferation and cytokine production. Splenocytes and hepatic lymph node cells cells from ALA-infected gerbils, for example, proliferated strongly to crude amebic proteins (AP) as early as 5 days after infection (21, 22). *E. histolytica* antigen-induced proliferation of peripheral blood mononuclear cells (PBMC) obtained from patients with active amebiasis was increased compared to controls (23). After pharmacologic cure of infection, PBMC from patients were found to proliferate and produce cytokines when stimulated with amebic antigen, demonstrating the development of antigen-specific memory (24, 25). Few of the peptide *E. histolytica* antigen recognized by T cells have been identified. Murine T cell clones have been raised against crude amebic proteins (26), but the specific antigens they recognized was not identified. The Gal-lectin, the most immunologically characterized amebic molecule, has recently been analysed for T cell epitopes. PBMC from patients with amebic dysentry or liver abscess proliferated in response to two different peptides of the Gal-lectin (27). Interestingly, the responses of dysentry patients were stronger than those of liver abscess patients, perhaps reflecting the immunosuppression associated with ALA.

Once activated, T cells may participate in an immune response against *E. histolytica* in three distinct ways: (1) by directly lysing amebas in a contact dependent manner; (2) by producing cytokines which activate macrophages (and possibly other effector cells) for amebicidal activity and; (3) by providing help for B cell antibody production.

Evidence of direct amebicidal activity by human T cells comes from a report by Salata and colleagues (26) in which the killing activity of phytohaemagglutinin (PHA)-stimulated T cells was examined. Incubation of amebas with PHA-activated T cells resulted in killing of 92% of the amebic trophozoites. This killing was contact- dependent and antibody-independent. In addition, the amoebicidal activity was abrogated by treatment of T cells with anti-OKT8 monoclonal antibody and complement, implicating CD8$^+$ T cells in the killing. Amebic proteins, as antigen, were also capable of activating T cells for amoebicidal activity, suggesting that this phenomenon may occur *in vivo*. T cells from ALA patients killed amebic trophozoites following 5 days stimulation with crude amebic antigen *in vitro* (24). Unstimulated T cells from ALA patients or control T cells stimulated with AP failed to kill *E. histolytica* trophoziotes. The parasite's immunodominant Gal-lectin has been identified as an amebic molecule that stimulates T cell amoebicidal activity. In a study of Gal-lectin-immunized gerbils, it was demonstrated that a 5-day incubation of gerbil spleen cells with Gal-lectin, followed by 6 hr co-incubation of these cells with amebas, resulted in amebic viability being reduced to 51.6% compared to controls (29). Under similar Gal-lectin stimulation and co-incubation conditions, PBMC from amebiasis patients reduced viability to 61% compared to controls (25).

The mechanism(s) by which T cells directly kill *E. histolytica*, trophoziotes was addressed in a study of amebic antigen-specific murine T cell clones (26). Two of 11 T cell clones generated from hyperimmunized mice were capable of directly killing amebas. At a 100 : 1 T cell/ameba ratio and after 6 hr co-incubation, the 2 antigen-activated CD8$^+$ T cell clones killed 76% and 86% of the amebas respectively. Supernatants of the activated clones did not kill amebas. However, addition of anti-TNF-α to the T cell clones prior to their interaction with amebas abrogated the killing. As exogenous TNF-α did not kill amebas, additional factors must have been involved. T cells have also been reported to kill fungal, bacterial and other parasite species *in vitro* in a direct, presumably major histocompatibility complex (MHC) un-restricted fashion (30). The mechanisms involved remain to be characterized.

There is considerable experimental evidence indicating that the major mechanism of T cell-mediated defence in amebiasis involves activation of macrophage for amoebicidal activity. Delayed-type hypersensitivity reactions to amebic antigen have been detected in both humans and animals (31, 32), indicating that cell-mediated immunity was activated in response to *E. histolytica in vivo*. In addition, several *in vitro* studies indicated that T cell-derived cytokines activate macrophages to kill amebas. A study using macrophages and T cells from uninfected humans demonstrated that supernatants from Concanavalin A (Con A), PHA, or amebic antigen-stimulated PBMC activated macrophages to kill 55% of the amebas within 3 hr (33). Supernatants of amebic antigen-stimulated PBMC from cured amebiasis patients also activated normal monocyte-derived macrophages to kill amebas (24). In addition, macrophages from these patients killed amebas when stimulated by supernatants of Con A-stimulated normal lymphocytes. Thus, macrophages and T cells of patients with a history of ALA were capable of co-operating in anti-amebic defence.

The identity of the T cell cytokine(s) involved in activating macrophage amoebicidal activity was addressed in a study of PBMC from patients with a history of amebiasis (34). It was demonstrated that normal macrophages activated with 300 U/ml of recombinant Interferon-γ (IFN-γ) killed 47% of co-incubated amebas in 6 hr. Stimulation of patient PBMC and normal PBMC with Con A resulted in equal levels of IFN-γ, but patient PBMC produced significantly more IFN-γ than normal PBMC when stimulated with amebic antigen (1,862 U/ml vs. 174 U/ml). Activation of normal macrophages with amebic antigen-stimulated patient PBMC supernatants resulted in killing of 48% of co-incubated amebas. This number was reduced to 18% killed in the presence of anti-IFN-γ antibodies, indicating that T cell-derived IFN-γ plays a major, but not exclusive, role in activating macrophages for amoebicidal activity. Other T cell-derived cytokines may be co-released with IFN-γ and participate in activating macrophages. Tumour necrosis factor-α/β (TNF-α/β) and Interleukin-2 (IL-2), for example, both have macrophage activating capacity (35, 36). IFN-γ and IL-2 were co-released from patient PBMC and from splenocytes of immune gerbils when cells were stimulated with the Gal-lectin in vitro (25, 29). Additionally, IL-2 and TNF-α were co-produced by amebic antigen-stimulated lymphoid cells isolated from gerbils with ALA (22).

Specific antigens may also stimulate T cell cytokine responses that downregulate macrophage-mediated defences. While peptides of a 220 kDa surface lectin of E. histolytica stimulated production of IL-2 and IFN-γ from lymphoid cells of mice immunized with the peptides, cells from mice immunized with the complete molecule produced IL-4 and IL-10 when stimulated in vitro (37). Both IL-4 and IL-10 act to suppress macrophage anti-microbial functions (38, 39). Hence, the type of T cell cytokine response may determine whether or not macrophages are activated for amoebicidal activity *in vitro*. These findings stress the importance of characterizing the immune responses stimulated by specific antigens being considered as vaccine candidates.

T cell cytokine responses have been divided into different classes based on the combination of cytokines produced. Th1 cytokine responses are characterized by T cell release of IL-2, IFN-γ and TNF-β, whereas Th2 cytokine responses are characterized by IL-4, -5, -6, -9 and -10 production and Th0 responses consist of a mix of Th1 and Th2 cytokines (40). Th1 responses tend to promote cell-mediated immunity (CMI) while Th2 responses are associated with humoral immunity (40). As the type of T cell response controls susceptibilty or resistance to infection in a number of infectious diseases, we recently examined IL-2 and IL-4 production from lymphoid cells of gerbils to determine the type of T cell responses operative during ALA development (22). Gerbil spleen and hepatic lymph node cells stimulated *ex vivo* with amebic antigen produced both IL-2 and IL-4 (Th0 response) early in infection (5 and 10 days post infection), whereas cytokine production was suppressed during the acute stage of the disease (20 days post infection). During late infection (30–60 days post infection), however, IL-2 production increased while IL-4 production remained low (Th1 response) (Fig. 1). In addition, gerbils drug-cured during acute infection were resistant to reinfection and also demonstrated Th1 responses (high IL-2 and low IL-4). These results suggested that a Th1 response, presumably resulting in cell-mediated immunity (CMI), was connected with resistance to ALA in gerbils.

The relentless progression of human hepatic amebiasis (41) may be the result of a failure to switch to a Th1 response during or following acute infection. As discussed above, cells from drug-cured patients produce high levels of the Th1 cytokines IL-2 and IFN-γ when stimulated *in vitro*. Although the cytokine responses of patients during active amebiasis have not been characterized, it is possible that drug-cure of these individuals allowed a switch to Th1 cytokine production, similar to what occurs in drug-cured gerbils.

T cells may also function in amebic infections by providing help for B cell antibody production (42). Although T cell help for B cells has not been directly studied in the context of amebiasis, antibodies are produced to several amebic antigens during infection (43). However, while anti-amebic IgG responses were detected in Balb/c mice injected with live amebas, nude (nu/nu) mice from a Balb/c background did not develop anti-amebic IgG

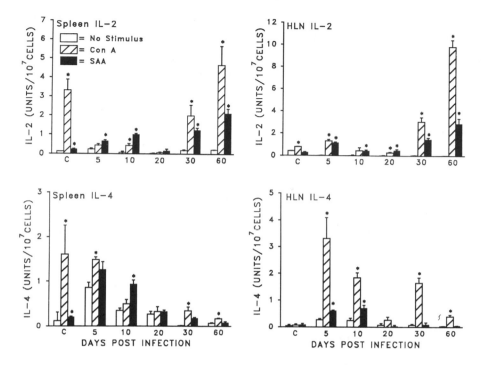

Figure 1. Kinetics of IL-2 and IL-4 production by spleen and hepatic lymph node (HLN) cells from gerbils with amoebic liver abscess and uninfected gerbils (C) in response to concanavalin A (Con A; 5 μg/well, 10^7 cells/well) or soluble amoebic antigen (SAA; 50 μg/well, 10^7 cells/well). Data are representative of duplicated experiments and are expressed as mean $\pm$ SE (4 wells/condition). * $P < 0.05$ vs. unstimulated homologous controls. (Reprinted with permission from *J. Infect. Dis.* **175**, 1176 (1997)).

responses to amebas (44). Thus, amebic antigen-specific T cells must act to promote antibody production, probably through cytokine release and contact-dependent stimulation of B cells.

Macrophage Responses

Evidence from *in vivo* and *in vitro* studies suggest that macrophage-mediated amoebicidal activity is a principal mode of host defence against invasive *E. histolytica* infections. Mechanisms of macrophage amoebicidal activity have been extensively characterized *in vitro*, more so than for other proposed modes of immunological defence against the parasite. Amebic molecules and host factors involved in macrophage activation and the cellular and molecular mechanisms employed by these effector cells in killing amebas have been identified and are reviewed below. *In vivo*, amebic antigen-specific activation of T cells, resulting in promotion of macrophage effector functions, should provide a rapid effector response limiting *E. histolytica* infections.

Injection of silica in hamsters resulted in functional depletion of macrophages as quantified by inhibited *ex vivo* macrophage phagocytosis (45). Consequently, the silica-treated hamsters experienced increased liver abscess size following direct hepatic inoculation of amebas. While nude mice were resistant to ALA, pretreatment with silica sensitized these animals to liver infection with *E. histolytica* (44). Additionally, pretreatment of hamsters with rabbit anti-macrophage serum, prior to inoculation with amebas, resulted in larger liver abscesses than pretreatment with normal rabbit serum (46). Therefore, *in vivo* treatments that knockout macrophages render animals susceptible to ALA or increased severity of infection, indicating the requirement for these cells in anti-amebic defence.

A variety of cytokines and microbial products have been shown to activate macrophages for amoebicidal activity *in vitro* (Table 1). In addition to the documented activation of macrophages by human T cell supernatants containing IFN-γ (34) and, presumably, other macrophage-activating cytokines, recombinant cytokines have been shown to activate macrophages to kill *E. histolytica* trophozoites *in vitro*. IFN-γ alone (100–1,000 U/ml) or in combination with 20–50 ng/ml bacterial lipopolysaccharide (LPS) activated murine bone marrow-derived macrophages (BMM) to kill 24–60% of amebas in a 6 hr assay (47). Macrophages isolated from mouse livers (Kupffer cells) also responded to IFN-γ and LPS stimulation by killing amebic trophozoites (48), suggesting that these tissue macrophages may be responsive during liver infections. Other cytokines such as colony-stimulating factor-1 (CSF-1) and TNF-α, alone or in synergy with IFN-γ, stimulated murine macrophage amoebicidal activity (47). *In vivo*, both TNF-β (produced by T cells) and TNF-α (produced by T cells and macrophages) may promote macrophage activation. *In vitro*, macrophage TNF-α acts in an autocrine fashion as a powerful activator of macrophage-mediated killing of amoebae (49). LPS and the cytokines IFN-γ and TNF-α have no direct cytotoxic effects on *E. histolytica* trophoziotes (47).

IFN-γ acts to prime macrophages for enhanced responsiveness to triggering signals (e.g. TNF-α) (50). Under certain conditions, transforming growth factor-β (TGF-β) further primed macrophages for amoebicidal activity

Table 1. Activation of macrophage amoebicidal activity by cytokines and LPS[a].

Stimulus (concentration)	Macrophage source [ref.]	% Amoebae killed
LPS (100 ng/ml)	murine bone marrow (54)	6
IFN-γ (300 U/ml)	human PBMC (34)	47
IFN-γ (100 U/ml)	murine bone marrow (47, 54)	24–55
IFN-γ (100 U/ml) + LPS (100Tng/ml)	murine bone marrow (49, 54)	66–72
IFN-γ (100 U/ml) + LPS (100 ng/ml)	gerbil peritonium (119)	40
TNF-α (100 U/ml)	murine bone marrow (47)	6
IFN-γ (100 U/ml) + TNF-α (100 U/ml)	murine bone marrow (47)	74
CSF-1 (10^4 U/ml)	murine bone marrow (47)	29
IFN-γ (10^3 U/ml) + CSF-1 (10^3 U/ml)	murine bone marrow (47)	83

[a]Macrophages in RPMI-1640 medium were pretreated with stimulants for 16–72 hr prior to co-incubation with *E. histolytica* trophozoites (100 : 1 ratio) at 37°C and 5% CO_2 for 6 hr. Viability was determined by trypan blue exclusion. Viability of amoebae co-incubated with naïve macrophages was 95–100%.

(51). Pretreatment of murine BMM for 4 hr with TGF-β primed these cells for a stimulated amebic killing response to IFN-γ + TNF-α or IFN-β + LPS (15% and 23% increases, respectively). This priming effect was highly dependent on the LPS (> 100 ng) or TNF-α (> 100 U) triggering dose in the presence of IFN-γ. At lower concentrations of LPS or TNF-α, TGF-β had a suppressive effect.

Following cytokine activation *in vitro*, macrophages kill *E. histolytica* trophozoites in a contact-dependent and antibody-independent manner (33, 47, 48). There is little evidence to support a role for macrophages in antibody-dependent cellular cytotoxicity (ADCC) in amebiasis (33, 52). In contrast, early reports suggested a role for reactive oxygen intermediates in macrophage amoebicidal activity. *E. histolytica* trophozoites are susceptible to exogenously added H_2O_2 (53). In addition, macrophage-mediated killing was partially inhibited by catalase but not superoxide dismutase, suggesting a role for H_2O_2 but not O_2^- in amoebicidal activity (33, 47). Representing a possible non-oxidative mechanism, the protease inhibitor tosyl-lysyl chlormethyl ketone inhibited amoebicidal activity by

61% (47). However, these studies did not fully account for the measured amoebicidal activity.

More recent studies have helped to clarify the mechanisms involved in macrophage-mediated killing of amebas. Lin and Chadee (54) found a correlation between murine macrophage nitric oxide (NO) production (measured as a stable end product: NO_2^-) and amoebicidal activity. Activation of elicited peritoneal macrophages (EPM) or BMM by a 24 hr pretreatment with IFN-γ (100 U/ml) + LPS (100 ng/ml) resulted in high NO production (18 μM $NO_2^-/10^6$ cells) and reduction of amebic viability from 97% to 26%. Macrophage-mediated amoebicidal activity was inhibited in a dose dependent fashion by arginase (Fig. 2) and N^G-monomethyl L-arginine (L-NMMA), which are inhibitors of L-arginine, the substrate for inducible nitric oxide synthase (iNOS). Incubation of *E. histolytica* trophozoites with NO-donors sodium nitrite or sodium nitroprusside further confirmed that amebas were susceptible to NO-mediated killing (54).

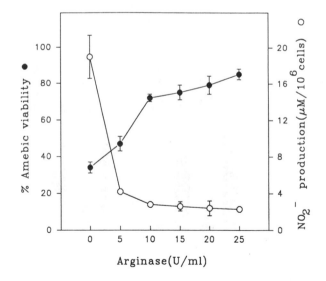

Figure 2. Inhibitory effects of arginase on NO_2^- production and amoebicidal activity of activated macrophages. Murine elicted peritoneal macrophages (2×10^6) were exposed to IFN-γ (100 U/ml) + LPS (100 ng/ml) in the presence of increasing concentrations of arginase for 24 hr before measuring NO_2^- production and amoebicidal activity. Data are means $\pm$ SD of duplicate experiments ($n = 8$). $p < 0.01$, compared with untreated (without arginase) controls. (Reprinted with permission from *J. Immunol.* **148**, 3999 (1992)).

Interestingly, H_2O_2 production did not correlate with amebic killing. Regardless of pretreatment conditions, phorbol myristate acetate (PMA)-triggered H_2O_2 levels were relatively constant, whereas pretreatment of macrophages with IFN-γ and LPS strongly augmented NO_2^- production and amoebicidal activity (Fig. 3). In addition, catalase was found to inhibit NO_2^- levels even at low concentrations (54). Catalase-inhibitable killing

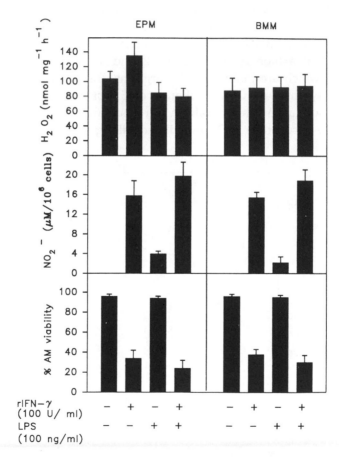

Figure 3. Relationship between amoebicidal activity and NO_2^- and H_2O_2 production by murine elicited peritoneal macrophages (EPM) and bone marrow-derived macrophages (BMM). Macrophages (2×10^6/ml) were exposed to IFN-γ alone or in combination with LPS for 24 hr before determining NO_2^- production, PMA-stimulated H_2O_2 release and amoebicidal activity. Data are means $\pm$ SD of triplicate experiments ($n = 10$). (Reprinted with permission from *J. Immunol.* **148**, 3999 (1992)).

attributed to H_2O_2 in previous studies may also have involved NO. However, it is possible that H_2O_2 may act as a co-factor or synergises with NO in amoebicidal activity. O_2^- may participate in the killing mediated by NO from L-arginine as well. Superoxide dismutase inhibited macrophage amoebicidal activity by 20% without affecting NO_2^- production (54).

Macrophage amoebicidal activity mediated by NO has been confirmed in subsequent studies (49, 55) and further investigation has revealed a key role for TNF-α in the upregulation of macrophage NO production. In IFN-γ + LPS stimulated macrophages L-NMMA inhibited NO_2^- production and amebic killing but had no effect on TNF-α production. However, anti-sera to TNF-α suppressed TNF-α release, NO_2^- production and amoebicidal activity by 93, 53 and 86%, respectively (49). Exogenous TNF-α, in combination with IFN-γ, also stimulated NO_2^- and amoebicidal activity. Macrophages stimulated with IFN-γ + TNF-α or LPS demonstrated enhanced levels of iNOS mRNA, peaking at 24 hr, and rapid expression of TNF-α mRNA, stable from 4 to 48 hr, concomitant with increased NO_2^- and TNF-α levels (49). Taken together, these data indicate that TNF-α is central for NO-dependent amoebicidal activity *via* elevated levels of iNOS mRNA expression, which may be associated with accumulation of TNF-α mRNA.

Cytokine stimulation of macrophage amoebicidal activity may be enhanced by *E. histolytica* components contributing to macrophage activation. Supporting this hypothesis is evidence of direct macrophage activation by amebic antigen. Injection of crude amoebic antigen in C57BL/6 mice followed by PMA-triggering of peritoneal exudate cells *in vitro* demonstrated that the antigen functioned to prime macrophages for enhanced respiratory burst activity compared to macrophages from saline-injected mice (56). Furthermore, pretreatment of EPM *in vitro* with partially purified low molecular weight amebic antigen primed these macrophages for enhanced PMA-triggered H_2O_2 and O_2^- release (57).

The Gal-lectin is, thus far, the only specific amebic molecule shown to directly stimulate macrophage functions. Murine BMM stimulated 3 hr with 500 ng Gal-lectin demonstrated an 8-fold increase in TNF-α mRNA expression and TNF-α protein production comparable to that of LPS (100 ng/ml)-stimulated BMM (58). A polyclonal anti-Gal-lectin serum inhibited TNF-α mRNA induction in response to Gal-lectin but not LPS. More specifically, anti-Gal-lectin mAbs 8C12, H85 and 1G7, which mapped to amino acids (aa) 596–1082 of the Gal-lectin 170 kDa subunit (59), inhibited both amebic adherence to mammalian cells and stimulation of TNF-α mRNA expression.

TNF-α mRNA expression in response to Gal-lectin was inhibited by 28, 82 and 84% respectively by mAbs 8C12, H85, 1G7 (Fig. 4).

Given that TNF-α was important in inducing macrophage NO production (49), a subsequent study examined the potential of Gal-lectin to stimulate macrophage iNOS mRNA expression and NO production (60). IFN-γ-primed murine BMM responded in a dose-dependent fashion to Gal-lectin with

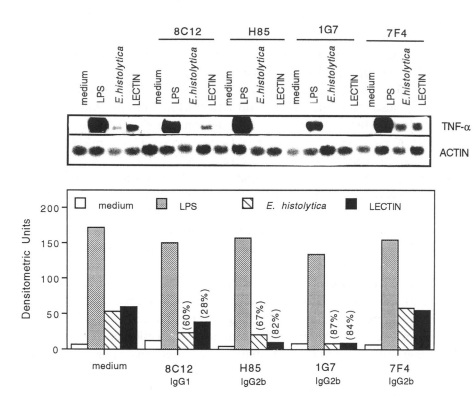

Figure 4. Anti-Gal-lectin mAbs inhibit TNF-α mRNA induction in murine bone-marrow-derived macrophages (BMM). LPS (100 ng/ml), soluble *E. histolytica* proteins (50 μg/ml), and purified Gal-lectin (100 ng/ml) were treated with either medium or affinity-purified mabs at 1 mg/ml for 1 hr at 4°C prior to incubation with macrophages for 1 hr at 37°C. Results of scanning densitometric analysis of Northern blot are presented as a histogram and are expressed as densitometric units with identical designations for blot lanes and histogram bars. Values in parentheses show percent inhibition of the response relative to BMMs in the presence of mab 7F4 or medium alone. (Reprinted with permission from *Proc. Natl. Acad. Sci. (USA)* **92**, 12175 (1995)).

increased levels of iNOS mRNA and NO_2^- production. In addition, IFN-γ + Gal-lectin stimulated macrophage amoebicidal activity (53% of amebas killed). Again, the stimulatory effect of Gal-lectin was specifically inhibited by mAb 1G7.

Neutrophil and Eosinophil Responses

E. histolytica produces a chemoattractant for neutrophils (61) and subsequently kills these cells on contact (62). Amebas also lyse unactivated monocytes/macrophages and eosinophils (33, 63). The lysis of polymorphonuclear neutrophils, in particular, has been associated with cell damage *in vivo* and *in vitro* due to the release of non-oxidative neutrophil toxins (5, 34, 64, 65). Despite the participation of neutrophils in tissue pathology, these effector cells, once activated, develop anti-amebic activity that may contribute to resistance to the parasite. Activation of human neutrophils with IFN-γ or IFN-γ + TNF-α rendered these cells more resistant to lysis by amebas and stimulated them to kill 30–60% amebas in a 6 hr *in vitro* assay (66). Physical separation of amebas and neutrophils by transwell membranes (0.45 μm) further augmented IFN-γ + TNF-α-stimulated neutrophil amoebicidal activity (up to 97% of the amebas were killed). Killing was inhibited 73% in the presence of catalase, leading the authors to conclude that H_2O_2 was the principal cytotoxic molecule. As human neutrophils also produce NO (67), which is inhibited by catalase (54), it is possible that neutrophil-derived NO could contribute to amoebicidal activity. *In vivo*, IFN-γ and TNF-α may act to promote both macrophage and neutrophil-mediated amoebicidal activity.

In SCID mice, depletion of neutrophils resulted in larger ALA at day 2 of infection (46.3% compared to 12.6% of liver abscessed) (68). The effect of neutrophil depletion was less marked by the seventh day of infection, suggesting that neutrophils may act early to inhibit abscess development. Other factors, independent of lymphocytes, may also contribute to control of infection in this model as SCID mice eventually resolve the infection (68).

A role for eosinophils in resistance to amebas is less clear. Eosinophils were activated for amoebicidal activity *in vitro* by treatment with f-Met-Leu-Phe (69) and eosinophilic infiltration of rat gut tissues occured in response to intragastric immunization with glutaraldehyde-fixed trophozoites (70). However, the *in vivo* relevence of eosinophil responses is unclear.

Humoral Responses

Seroepidemiologic studies indicate that 81% to 100% of patients with invasive amebiasis develop specific circulatory antibodies against *E. histolytica* (71). High titre serum antibody responses to *E. histolytica* were detectable within 7 days of infection (72) and a wide variety of *E. histolytica* antigens reacted with these antibodies (73). Major amebic antigens include the serine-rich *E. histolytica* protein (SREHP), which was recognized by sera of more than 80% of amebiasis patients (74) and was protective against ALA in gerbils (75). Similarily, the Gal-lectin and a 29 kDa amebic surface antigen are immunodominant amebic molecules and were protective in gerbils (76, 77). The Gal-lectin reacted with up to 95% of serum samples taken from different geographical locations (76, 78).

E. histolytica initiates infection at the intestinal mucosal surface and first encounters humoral responses at this site. Accordingly, the secretory antibody response at different mucosal sites has been investigated by a number of workers. Secretory anti-amebic IgA (sIgA) has been detected in the bile of intra-caecally-immunized rats (79) and in the faeces of amebiasis patients (80). sIgA responses against amebas are present at other mucosal sites as well. Anti-amebic sIgA has been detected in human milk (81) and saliva (80, 82).

Apart from serum (80) and secretory IgA, the dominant class of antibodies produced against *E. histolytica* appears to be IgG (71). Both the Gal-lectin and SREHP molecules, for example, stimulated strong serum IgG responses in immunized animals (76, 83). Serum IgM has been detected in human cases of intestinal and extra-intestinal disease (84, 85), whereas IgE may be produced during amebiasis but definitive reports are rare (70). How the humoral response relates to development of CMI is unclear. Th1 and Th2-type responses are linked to production of specific antibody subclasses (86). The frequencies of different antibody subclasses in amebiasis remain to be investigated.

While the development of antibody responses accompanies infection or follows immunization, these responses have not been considered protective in amebiasis (71, 87). Antibody titres do not correlate with resistance to infection in either clinical disease or animal models (82, 88–90). In patients, intestinal colonization with *E. histolytica* and progressive amebiasis appear to be uninhibited by high antibody titres (72, 91). Antibody responses may merely be an indication of current or recent invasive disease (80).

Recent reports have demonstrated various levels of protection against intra-hepatic challenge with amebas following passive immunization of immunologically incompetent SCID mice with anti-*E. histolytica* sera or purified antibodies or with anti-sera against the Gal-lectin or SREHP molecules (6, 90, 92, 93). Recently, immunization with a polypeptide of the cysteine-rich region (r170CR2) of Gal-lectin protected 62.5% of gerbils from ALA (90). Interestingly, a 25 amino acid (aa) peptide derived from r170CR2 was only recognized by the sera of gerbils protected following immunization with r170CR2. Sera of gerbils unsuccessfully immunized with r170CR2 did not react with this peptide (90). Hence, this peptide appeared to be immunoprotective. However, the fact that serum antibodies of some gerbils and of a r170CR2-immunized rabbit did not recognize the 25 aa peptide (90) suggests that genetic restriction may limit its usefulness as a vaccine candidate. In contrast to studies in SCID mice, passive immunization with various concentrations of ammonium sulphate-precipitated anti-amebic antibodies from rabbits or hamsters failed to protect immunologically competent hamsters from ALA (94).

Whereas key mechanisms used by macrophages in killing ameba have been identified (49, 54), how passive transfer of antibodies protects SCID mice from subsequent intra-hepatic challenge with *E. histolytica* remains to be demonstrated. *In vitro*, murine mAbs to the Gal-lectin molecule inhibited *E. histolytica* complement resistance (15) and adherence of amebas to cells (95), a necessary prerequisite for cytolysis of target cells (8, 96). Several reports of protective immunization in animals have suggested a link between protection and the presence of antibodies shown to have adherence-inhibitory effects *in vitro* (89, 97, 98). Human anti-amebic antibodies have also been shown to inhibit adherence to target cells *in vitro* (99, 100). However, these *in vitro* adherence assays were generally performed at 4°C (89, 90). At 37°C amebas capped and released or ingested antibodies bound to their surface (101, 102). *E. histolytica* produces a neutral cysteine protease which degraded human serum and secretory IgA (103). Purified amebic neutral cysteine protease cleaved IgG as well, reducing binding of IgG to amebas by 80% (104). Antibodies bound to the surface of *E. histolytica* may not last long enough to have significant effects.

If antibodies were to mediate resistance to amebas, activation of complement-mediated killing of trophozoites would be a possible mechanism. However, there is little complement in the gut (105) and IgA, which persists in the gut for a short time in amebiasis (106), does not fix complement (107). In serum, IgG fixation of complement is unlikely to play a major role given the parasite's resistance to complement-mediated lysis (15). A role for antibodies in eosinophil or neutrophil ADCC against amebas has not been demonstrated, while macrophages have been shown not to participate in ADCC against amebas (33, 52). Taken together, data demonstrate that amebas are resistant to the principal antibody-mediated defence mechanisms.

Possibly, antibodies contribute to resistance through transient agglutination of trophozoites that are subsequently dealt with by other mechanisms. Non-specific effects of passively transferred antibodies also can not be ruled out. SCID mice resolve amebic liver infections spontaneously in the absence of antibodies (68). Therefore, antibodies are not required for control of infection. Studies in nude mice confirm this. Nude mice failed to develop antibody responses to injected amebas whereas their thymus-intact littermates did (44). Nonetheless, nude mice were resistant to ALA unless depleted of macrophages by silica treatment (44). In SCID mice, which have functional natural killer (NK) cells and macrophages, NK cell activation of macrophages has been identified as an important mechanism controlling microbial infections (108) and may play a role in limiting ALA in these mice.

Apart from a possible contribution to resistance or control of infection, limited reports suggest that anti-amebic antibodies may have deleterious consequences and exacerbate disease. Antibodies to the Gal-lectin have been shown to enhance adherence of trophozoites to target cells (109), which may result in increased pathology due to elevated killing of host cells. In one study of amebiasis patients, immune complexes, which may contribute to pathogenesis (71), were detected in patient colonic (71 of 122 patients) and liver tissue (5 of 16 patients) (110). Sera from some amebiasis patients were shown to contain antibodies that block binding of anti-Ia mAbs to T cells and inhibited autologous mixed lymphocyte reactions (111). If this phenomenon occurs *in vivo*, suppression of antigen-specific immunity may result.

Amebic Modulation of Host Resistance Mechanisms

A complex interaction occurs between host cells and amebas during hepatic infections. *E. histolytica* rapidly kills naïve macrophages, T cells and neutrophils on contact (33). Amebas are also capable of modulating several T cell and macrophage responses during active infection (112). Specifically, the acute phase of hepatic amebiasis in humans and in animal models is associated with a transient state of immunosuppression, favouring amebic survival (21, 113, 114). Overcoming amebic immunomodulatory effects is probably key to controlling the infection. The fact that suppression appears to be transient suggests that, in some cases, the host may eventually be able to reverse the modulatory effects, but how this occurs is unclear.

Active infection is associated with T cell hyporesponsiveness as quantified by *in vitro* proliferative responses of patient T cells to mitogens Con A and PHA (23, 24). Hence, invasive amebiasis is associated with reduced T cell numbers (115). Depressed delayed-type hypersensitivity (DTH) reactions during acute disease (113) may be a sign of reduced T cell numbers and/ or inhibited development of antigen-specific immunity. In gerbils, T cell proliferation and cytokine release in response to Con A and amebic antigen are suppressed during acute infection (day 20) but recovered at days 30–60 of infection (22). Injection of amebic antigen in mice also resulted in depressed proliferative responses to mitogen (116). Involvement of a soluble factor, either an amebic molecule(s) or factor produced by the host in response to amebas, is suggested by the inhibitory effect of patient sera on antigen-specific T cell proliferation and IFN-γ production (117). The inhibitory effect of patient sera decreased as time between drug therapy and collection of sera increased (117). The apparent switch from a Th0 to Th1 response following acute disease in gerbils (22) may be a crucial step in controlling infection. A Th1-like response was also evident following drug-cure or immunization of gerbils (22, 29) and in drug-cured humans (25). Drug-cure, resulting in the removal of the parasite and associated suppressive effects, may have allowed the development of Th1 macrophage-activating responses.

During hepatic amebiasis, macrophages in the vicinity of the amebic abscess may be profoundly suppressed in several key accessory and effector functions while those distal from the abscess are in a heightened state of activation (21). This suggests that macrophage suppression in amebiasis is principally a local event mediated by direct exposure to amebas or amebic products, a hypothesis supported by the *in vitro* modulatory effects of amebic antigen on naïve macrophages. Liver-abscess-derived macrophages produced low basal levels of TNF-α that may contribute to abscess development (118). However, pretreatment of naïve macrophages with amebic antigen *in vitro* inhibited LPS- or IFN-γ + LPS-stimulated TNF-α gene expression and protein production. This could partially be accounted for induction of macrophage prostaglandin-E_2 (PGE$_2$) production (118, 119). *E. histolytica* also suppressed macrophage IL-1 production by an unknown mechanism (21). Significantly, ALA is associated with modulation of macrophage effector molecules and amebicidal activity. Abscess-derived macrophages were found to be hyporesponsive to PMA-triggered H_2O_2 production (21), and IFN-γ + LPS stimulation for NO production and amoebicidal activity (119). *In vitro*, pretreatment of naïve macrophages with amebic antigen suppressed iNOS mRNA expression, NO production and amoebicidal activity *via* a PGE_2-independent mechanism (119). Macrophages *in vivo* would not only be inhibited by low production of activating cytokines from T cells during acute infection, but also by suppressed ability to respond to activating signals for amebic killing. Macrophages may be partially responsible for weak T cell activation. Pretreatment of naïve macrophages *in vitro* with whole soluble amebic antigen or secreted products from trophozoites downregulated macrophage I-Aβ mRNA accumulation and surface Ia molecule expression in response to IFN-γ (120). The effect of amebic antigen on Ia expression was partially inhibited by indomethacin, indicating a role for PGE_2 in suppression of macrophage Ia expression (120). Reduced Ia expression could inhibit macrophage antigen-presenting cell capability resulting in the suppression of antigen-specific activation of T cells.

Sensitization of the immune system resulting from immunization or as a consequence of drug-termination of infection appears to be sufficient for the host to overcome the suppressive effects of *E. histolytica*, as evidenced by protection against parasite challenge. Paradoxically, the suppression of CMI associated with acute infection may support the concept of macrophage-mediated resistance being central to controlling invasive amebiasis. However, while gerbils may control the infection by switching to a Th1 macrophage-activating response, humans may not be able to affect this switch (assuming the pattern of gerbil T cell responses is paralleled in humans) in the absence of drug-cure.

Summary and Future Considerations

The interaction between *E. histolytica* and the host immune system is an intricate interplay involving elements of innate and acquired immune defences and modulation of these defences by the parasite. Immunization studies in animal models of the disease and limited epidemiological studies indicate that the senstized host may overcome the modulatory effects of amebas and mount a successful defence against invasive infection. Taken together, the experimental data reviewed above outline the mechanisms by which this resistance to *E. histolytica* is achieved.

In vitro studies have shown macrophages to be potent effector cells for amoebicidal activity and have demonstrated precise mechanisms involved. *In vivo*, functional elimination of these cells enables ALA to develop or significantly exacerbates the disease; and suppression of macrophages is associated with the acute stage of infection. Investigation of T cell responses indicates that drug-cured patients and drug-curedor immunized animals exhibit Th-1 macrophage-activating responses *ex vivo*. While more studies are required to conclusively prove that drug-cured patients are resistant to reinfection, animals, drug-cured or immunized, are resistant to invasive amebiasis and this resistance is linked to T cell/macrophage-mediated amoebicidal activity *in vitro*.

In contrast, development of antibody responses does not correlate with protection in patients or animal models. Studies in immunodeficient SCID mice have shown that passive transfer of antibodies is associated with protection against subsequent intra-hepatic challenge with *E. histolytica* trophozoites. However, the mechanism of protection has not been demonstrated and these studies have not been reproduced in immunocompetent animals. While amebic-induced suppression of macrophages during acute disease may be reversed, *E. histolytica*'s innate defences against antibodies are, presumably, always operative. Polymorphonuclear cells can be activated to demonstrate amoebicidal activity *in vitro*, but these cells have also been implicated in the tissue pathology associated with invasive amebiasis and their role in anti-amebic defence is unclear.

Many aspects of the interaction between *E. histolytica* and host humoral and CMI responses warrant further investigation. The susceptibility of SCID mice to ALA provides a useful tool to examine the roles of humoral and cellular responses. The development of ALA in these animals may be the result of antibody deficiency and/or lack of T cell-stimulated CMI. SCID/beige mice are deficient in B, T and NK cells, the latter being a source of IFN-γ for macrophage activation. Perhaps these mice have more prolonged infections compared to SCID mice. Gerbils are the principal immuno competent model of amebiasis (5) and the recent cloning of cytokine genes in these animals should enable more detailed analysis of cytokine responses during ALA. In humans with active disease, analysis of cytokine gene expression and production by PBMC cells and of the antibody subclasses produced during infection should further illuminate the types of immune responses that develop during amebiasis.

The development of a vaccine against *E. histolytica* should be a priority. Animal studies demonstrate the feasibility of vaccination to prevent infection and the pathology and immunosuppression associated with invasive disease. The immunodominant Gal-lectin, for example, would be a good vaccine candidate as it has been shown to contain both B and T cell epitopes and contributed to macrophage activation.

Acknowledgements

Research presented in this chapter from the author's laboratory was supported by the Natural Sciences and Engineering Research Council of Canada and the Medical Research Council of Canada. Research at the Institute of Parasitology is supported by the Fonds pour la Formation de Chercheurs et l'Aide à la Recherche du Quebéc (FCAR). Darren Campbell is the recipient of a PhD studentship from FCAR.

References

1. Walsh JA (1986). *Rev. Infect. Dis.* **8**: 228.
2. De Leon A (1970). *Arch. Invest. Med.* **1**: s205.
3. Petri Jr WA (1996). *Crit. Rev. Clin. Lab. Sci.* **33**: 1.
4. Stanley Jr SL (1996). *Parasitol. Today* **12**: 7.
5. Chadee K and Meerovitch E (1984). *Am. J. Pathol.* **117**: 71.
6. Cieslak RP, *et al.* (1992). *J. Exp. Med.* **176**: 1605.
7. Mai Z, *et al.* (1994). *Vet. Immunol. Immunopathol.* **40**: 63.
8. Chadee K, *et al.* (1987). *J. Clin. Invest.* **80**: 1245.
9. Chadee K, *et al.* (1991). *Gastroenterology* **100**: 986.
10. Ravdin JI (1989). *Pathol. Immunopathol. Res.* **8**: 179.
11. Calderon J and Schreiber RD (1985). *Infect. Immun.* **50**: 560.
12. Capin R, *et al.* (1980). *Arch. Invest. Med. (Mex)* **11 (s1)**: 173.
13. Calderon J and Tovar R (1986). *Immunology* **58**: 467.
14. Reed SL, *et al.* (1986). *J. Immunol.* **136**: 2265.
15. Braga LL, *et al.* (1992). *J. Clin. Invest.* **90**: 1131.
16. Desai AC and Bhide MB (1977). *Bull. Hoff. Inst.* **5**: 35.
17. Ghadirian E and Meerovitch E (1981). *Parasite Immunol.* **3**: 329.
18. Vinayak VK, *et al.* (1982). *Ann. Trop. Med. Hyg.* **76**: 309.
19. Ghadirian E, *et al.* (1987). *Trop. Med. Parasit.* **38**: 153.
20. Ghadirian E and Meerovitch E (1983). *Parasite Immunol.* **5**: 369.
21. Denis M and Chadee K (1988). *Infect. Immun.* **56**: 3126.
22. Campbell D and Chadee K (1997). *J. Infec. Dis.* **175**: 1176.

23. Simjee AE, *et al.* (1985). *Trans. R. Soc. Trop. Med. Hyg.* **79**: 165.
24. Salata RA, *et al.* (1986). *J. Immunol.* **136**: 2633.
25. Schain DC, *et al.* (1992). *Infect. Immun.* **60**: 2143.
26. Denis M and Chadee K (1989). *Immunology* **66**: 76.
27. Velazquez C, *et al.* (1995). *J. Euk. Microbiol.* **42**: 636.
28. Salata RA, *et al.* (1987). *Parasite Immunol.* **9**: 249.
29. Schain DC, *et al.* (1995). *J. Parasitol.* **81**: 563.
30. Levitz SM, *et al.* (1995). *Immunol. Today* **16**: 387.
31. Kretschmer RR, *et al.* (1972). *Trop. Georg. Med.* **24**: 275.
32. Gold D (1989). *Parasitol. Res.* **75**: 335.
33. Salata RA, *et al.* (1985). *J. Clin. Invest.* **76**: 491.
34. Salata RA, *et al.* (1987). *Am. J. Trop. Med. Hyg.* **37**: 72.
35. Nacy CA, *et al.* (1990). *Pathobiology* **59**: 182.
36. Espinoza-Delgado I, *et al.* (1995). *J. Leukoc. Biol.* **57**: 13.
37. Talamas-Rohana P, *et al.* (1995). *Infect. Immun.* **63**: 3953.
38. Taub DD and Cox GW (1995). *J. Leukoc. Biol.* **58**: 80.
39. Reiner SL (1994). *Immunol. Today* **15**: 374.
40. Mosmann TR and Sad S (1996). *Immunol. Today* **17**: 138.
41. Adams EB and MacLeod IN (1977). *Medicine (Baltimore)* **56**: 325.
42. Noelle RJ and Snow EC (1991). *FASEB J.* **5**: 2770.
43. Joyce MP and Ravdin JI (1988). *Am. J. Trop. Med. Hyg.* **38**: 74.
44. Stern JJ, *et al.* (1984). *Am. J. Trop. Med. Hyg.* **33**: 372.
45. Ghadirian E and Meerovitch E (1982). *Parasite Immunol.* **4**: 219.
46. Ghadirian E, *et al.* (1983). *Infect. Immun.* **42**: 1017.
47. Denis M and Chadee K (1989). *Infect. Immun.* **57**: 1750.
48. Ghadirian E and Salimi A (1993). *Immunobiol.* **188**: 203.
49. Lin JY, *et al.* (1994). *Infect. Immun.* **62**: 1534.
50. Krammer PH, *et al.* (1985). *J. Immunol.* **135**: 3258.
51. Lin JY, *et al.* (1995). *Immunology* **85**: 400.
52. Saxena A and Vinayak VK (1987). *Trans. R. Soc. Trop. Med. Hyg.* **81**: 933.
53. Murray HW, *et al.* (1981). *Mol. Biochem. Parasitol.* **3**: 381.
54. Lin JY and Chadee K (1992). *J. Immunol.* **148**: 3999.
55. Denis M and Ghadirian E (1992). *Microbial Pathogenesis* **12**: 193.
56. Ghadirian E and Kongshavn PAL (1988). *Microbial Pathogenesis* **5**: 63.
57. Lin JY, *et al.* (1993). *Immunology* **78**: 291.
58. Séguin R, *et al.* (1995). *Proc. Natl. Acad. Sci. (USA)* **92**: 12175.
59. Mann BJ, *et al.* (1993). *Infect. Immun.* **61**: 1772.
60. Séguin R, *et al.* (1997). *Infect. Immun.* **65**: 2522.

61. Salata RA, *et al.* (1989). *J. Parasitol.* **75**: 644.

62. Guerrant RL, *et al.* (1981). *J. Infect. Dis.* **143**: 83.

63. Lopez-Osuna M and Kretschmer RR (1989). *Parasite Immunol.* **11**: 403.

64. Tsutsumi V, *et al.* (1984). *Am. J. Pathol.* **117**: 81.

65. Salata RA and Ravdin JI (1986). *J. Infect. Dis.* **154**: 19.

66. Denis M and Chadee K (1989). *J. Leuk. Biol.* **46**: 270.

67. Evans TJ, *et al.* (1996). *Proc. Natl. Acad. Sci. (USA)* **93**: 9553.

68. Seydel KB, *et al.* (1997). *Infect Immun.* **65**: 3951.

69. Lopez-Osuna M, *et al.* (1992). *Parasite Immunol.* **14**: 579.

70. Navarro-Garcia F, *et al.* (1997). *Clin. Immunol. Immunopath.* **82**: 221.

71. Salata RA and Ravdin JI (1986). *Rev. Infect. Dis.* **8**: 261.

72. Katzenstein D, *et al.* (1982). *Medicine* **61**: 237.

73. Ximenez C, *et al.* (1992). *Ann. Trop. Med. Parasitol.* **86**: 121.

74. Stanley Jr SL (1991). *JAMA* **266**: 1984.

75. Zhang T, *et al.* (1994). *Infect. Immun.* **62**: 1166.

76. Soong C-JG, *et al.* (1995). *J. Infect. Dis.* **171**: 645.

77. Soong C-JG, *et al.* (1995). *Infect. Immun.* **63**: 472.

78. Petri Jr WA, *et al.* (1989). *Am. J. Med. Sci.* **296**: 163.

79. Acosta G, *et al.* (1983). *Ann. N.Y. Acad. Sci.* **409**: 760.

80. Abou-El-Magd I, *et al.* (1996). *J. Infect. Dis.* **174**: 157.

81. Grundy MS, *et al.* (1983). *J. Clin. Microbiol.* **17**: 753.

82. Kelsall BL, *et al.* (1994). *Am. J. Trop. Med. Hyg.* **51**: 454.

83. Zhang T, *et al.* (1995). *Infect. Immun.* **63**: 1349.

84. Harris WG and Bray RS (1976). *Trans. R. Soc. Trop. Med. Hyg.* **70**: 340.

85. Schulz TF, *et al.* (1987). *Trop. Med Parasitol.* **38**: 149.

86. Mosmann TR and Coffman RL (1989). *Ann. Rev. Immunol.* **7**: 145.

87. Jackson TFHG (1985). *Lancet* **2**: 716.

88. Krupp IM (1970). *Am. J. Trop. Med.* **19**: 57.

89. Petri Jr WA and Ravdin JI (1991). *Infect. Immun.* **59**: 97.

90. Lotter H, *et al.* (1997). *J. Exp. Med.* **185**: 1793.

91. Irusen EM, *et al.* (1992). *Clin. Infect. Dis.* **14**: 889.

92. Seydel KB, *et al.* (1996). *Am. J. Trop. Med. Hyg.* **55**: 330.

93. Zhang T, *et al.* (1994). *Parasite Immunol.* **16**: 225.

94. Campos-Rodriguez R, *et al.* (1995). *Parasitol. Res.* **81**: 86.

95. Ravdin JI, *et al.* (1986). *Infect. Immun.* **53**: 1.

96. Ravdin JI and Guerrant RL (1981). *J. Clin. Invest.* **68**: 1305.

97. Beving DE, *et al.* (1996). *Infect. Immun.* **64**: 1473.

98. Kelsall BL and Ravdin JI (1995). *Infect. Immun.* **63**: 686.

99. Carrero JC, *et al.* (1994). *Infect. Immun.* **62**: 764.

100. Petri Jr WA, *et al.* (1987). *Infect. Immun.* **55**: 2327.

101. Calderon J, *et al.* (1980). *J. Exp. Med.* **151**: 184.

102. Espinosa-Cantellano M and Martinez-Palomo A (1994). *Exp. Parasitol.* **79**: 424.

103. Kelsall BL and Ravdin JI (1993). *J. Infect. Dis.* **168**: 1319.

104. Herdman DS, *et al.* (1997). *Arch. Med. Res.* **28**: s178.

105. Kilian M and Russell MW (1994). *Handbook of Mucosal Immunology*, eds. Ogra PL, *et al.* (Academic Press, San Diego).

106. Martinez-Cairo CS, *et al.* (1979). *Arch. Invest. Med. (Mex.)* **10**: 121.

107. Liszewski MK and Atkinson JP (1993). *Fundamental Immunology*, ed. Paul WE (Raven Press, New York).

108. Bancroft GJ, *et al.* (1991). *Immunological Rev.* **124**: 5.

109. Petri Jr WA, *et al.* (1990). *J. Immunol.* **144**: 4803.

110. Mukherjee RM, *et al.* (1994). *Trans. R. Soc. Trop. Med. Hyg.* **88**: 546.

111. De Simone C, *et al.* (1984). *Trans. R. Soc. Trop. Med. Hyg.* **78**: 64.

112. Campbell D and Chadee K (1997). *Parasitol. Today* **13**: 184.

113. Ortiz-Ortiz L, *et al.* (1975). *Clin. Immunol. Immunopathol.* **4**: 127.

114. Gill NJ, *et al.* (1985). *Trans. Roy. Soc. Trop. Med. Hyg.* **79**: 618.

115. Gandhi BM, *et al.* (1986). *J. Trop. Med. Hyg.* **89**: 163.

116. Chadee K, *et al.* (1991). *Parasitol. Res.* **77**: 572.

117. Salata RA, *et al.* (1990). *Infect. Immun.* **58**: 3941.

118. Wang W, *et al.* (1992). *Infect. Immun.* **60**: 3169.

119. Wang W, *et al.* (1994). *Immunology* **83**: 601.

120. Wang W and Chadee K (1995). *Infect. Immun.* **63**: 1089.

Chapter 4

Pathogenesis and Molecular Biology

G Ramakrishan and WA Petri, Jr

Room 2115 MR4 Building, Lane Road
University of Virginia HSC, Charlottesville, VA 22908, USA
E-mail: gr6q@virginia.edu, wap3g@virginia.edu

The ability of the *E. histolytica* trophozoite to invade the colon and other tissues, and to persist in the face of the host immune response depends upon adaptation and expression of pathogenic factors. These pathogenic factors control the capabilities for extracellular matrix destruction, contact-dependent cytolysis of host tissue, and development of complement resistance, which are important aspects of invasion. Transcriptional regulation of virulence factors may be an important mechanism for modulating the pathogenic potential of the parasite. This chapter presents the known molecular aspects of transcription and pathogenesis, focusing on the best characterized virulence factors of *E. histolytica*.

Introduction

Infection by *E. histolytica* may result in asymptomatic colonisation of the large bowel, or it may lead to symptomatic disease. Invasion past the mucous barrier of the colonic epithelium leads to the development of colitis and amebic dysentery. Dissemination of the trophozoite through the blood stream permits the invasion of other tissues, most frequently the liver, resulting in abscesses in these extracolonic locations. The ability of the trophozoite to survive, and indeed, to flourish in these varied environments is indicative of the adaptability of the parasite. The trophozoite undergoes encystation in the bowel, generating cysts. The cysts are heat resistant, acid-stable, and propagate the infection by oral-fecal spread. Excystation in the bowel of a new host releases new trophozoites that can establish infection.

While much about the factors governing these various aspects of pathogenesis by the organism remains to be determined, some advances have been made in understanding the determinants that make it a successful parasite. Probing the genetic make-up and the molecular biology of the organism will help both to understand what causes pathogenicity, and how it may be successfully overcome. The molecular biological approach is particularly compelling because it has provided the first tools to conclusively distinguish *E. histolytica* from the morphologically similar, but non-pathogenic species, *E. dispar*, and thereby should permit identification of those mechanisms that are specific to pathogenicity.

The nature of the *E. histolytica* genome has been discussed in detail by Clark *et al.* (Sec. 2). The DNA is A + T rich, with a total G + C content of 25% (1). The G + C content of coding regions is 33%, with 16% in the third position (2, 3). Gene organization in *E. histolytica* is quite different from that in higher eukaryotes. As may be expected for a small genome, genes are closely linked with intergenic distances less than 1.5 kb for three structural genes examined (4). Two genes with no intergenic gap whatever have recently been described; the 3' end of the *pak* RNA shares a 40 base overlap with the 5' end of the *mcm3* RNA (5). Analysis of most protein-coding genes from *E. histolytica* shows that the 5' untranslated regions of mRNAs are unusually short (5–21 bases) as are the 3' untranslated regions (14–61 bases) (4). Only a few genes have been reported to have long untranslated regions at their 5' or 3' ends (5–7). There is evidence for capping of at least one mRNA (8). mRNA splicing is rare; only three genes have been shown to contain introns, all of which are small (7, 9, 10). The existence of conventional splicing machinery is indicated by the isolation of the gene encoding the u6 small nuclear RNA (11). There is no evidence of trans-splicing or polycistronic transcription (4).

Transcription of protein-encoding genes in *E. histolytica* is resistant to α-amanitin (12), in contrast to RNA polymerase II from higher eukaryotes. This may reflect the variant structure of the *E. histolytica* polymerase II subunit, analogous to that of another early divergent protozoan with α-amanitin resistant RNA polymerase II, *Trichomonas vaginalis* (13).

In contrast to most metazoan cells, the rDNA genes of *E. histolytica* are carried on circular plasmids rather than on linear chromosomes. Present in 200 copies per genome in the strain HM-1 : IMSS, the 24.5 kb rDNA episome is the best characterized DNA molecule in *E. histolytica* (14–16). It has been adopted as a model for the study of replication in the organism. A region of the rDNA episome containing a family of 170 bp repeats was shown to confer replicating ability in yeast when cloned into a yeast plasmid lacking autonomous replication consensus sequences (17). The technique of neutral/neutral two-dimensional gel electrophoresis was used to examine replication initiation in the rDNA episome (18). In contrast to plasmids in other eukaryotic and bacterial systems, replication in the amebic plasmid was found to initiate at multiple sites with no sequence specificity, and the majority of the origins appeared to lie within the rDNA transcribed region (18). The apparent lack of sequence specificity may result from the A – T richness of the amebic genome. The link to transcription may reflect the imposition of a control mechanism on an otherwise unregulated event; DNA replication could be controlled by the rate of transcription that, in turn, is controlled by the metabolic state of the cell. The study of replication in *E. histolytica* is still in its infancy, but the ability to transfect engineered DNA into the trophozoite (19–21) should provide new avenues for further analysis of replication and replication factors.

Although conventional eukaryotic structures associated with protein synthesis and trafficking, such as rough endoplasmic reticulum and Golgi bodies, have not been observed in the trophozoite, the existence of several secreted and membrane-associated proteins (22–34), with precursors possessing signal peptides, indicates that a secretory pathway is functional in *E. histolytica*. The homologue of the 54 kDa subunit of the eukaryotic signal recognition particle (SRP54) has been identified (8), indicating conservation of the secretion machinery. Glycosylation (N- and O-linked) and acylation, and addition of glycosylphosphatidylinositol anchors, functions that are associated with trafficking organelles — the ER and the Golgi bodies, are also observed on amebic proteins (33, 35, 36). The best characterized pathogenic factors, the Gal/GalNAc lectin, the amoebapores and the cysteine proteinases are all dependent on transport through the secretory pathway.

Transcriptional Control

There is great variability in virulence characteristics of different isolates of *E. histolytica*. Virulence of trophozoites is also influenced by external factors such as animal passage (37–39), growth in the presence of cholesterol (38, 40), and exposure to certain bacteria (41, 42). Thus environmental factors play a role in regulating pathogenicity, and it is reasonable to suppose that, analogous to other well-characterized systems of prokaryotes and higher eukaryotes, primary control over the invasive capability of the parasite is exerted at the level of gene expression. Variation in specific mRNA levels has been observed following changes in conditions of growth; superoxide dismutase gene expression is induced by superoxide radical anions (43), the EhADH2 gene, encoding alcohol/aldehyde dehydrogeanase, is induced by ethanol (44), actin gene expression has been shown to be autoregulated (45), and ferredoxin gene expression has been shown to be growth-sensitive (46). The acquisition of resistance to emetine has been shown to be related to increased expression of the P-glycoprotein mRNA (47). While the process of encystation has not yet been successfully accomplished in laboratory cultures of *E. histolytica*, it can be studied in the species of *Entamoeba invadens*; encysting *E. invadens* parasites show increased levels of certain mRNAs, including those for chitinases (34, 48, 49). Differential gene expression may therefore be a significant factor controlling pathogenicity of the trophozoite, including processes of invasion, encystation and excystation, and adaptation to the aerobic environment of human tissues following invasion.

In order to determine how genes may be differentially regulated, it is important to first understand the basic promoter architecture of the amebic gene. Several elements controlling gene expression have been identified in different gene promoters (4, 43, 50–52). With the advent of transient transfection (19–21) and stable transfection (53, 54) techniques, the detailed analysis of gene expression at the molecular level has become feasible. In our lab, work has largely focused on understanding the control of transcription at the promoter of the lectin gene, *hgl5*. Initial studies showed that 1.0 kb of the 5' flanking DNA from the *hgl5* gene could direct specific transcription of a reporter gene on an episome (20). In a further detailed analysis of the promoter structure, the promoter was narrowed down to 272 bp upstream of the transcription start, and mutational analysis led to the identification of five Upstream Regulatory Elements (URE) in addition to the conserved core promoter elements directing transcription (51) (Fig. 1). Both negative and positive control elements were identified. The URE1 and URE2 elements contain homology to higher eukaryotic activator elements; PEA3 sequence homology is found in both of the URE elements, while URE2 also shows homology to the AP-1 element (51). Although URE1 and URE2 were shown to be positive elements regulating gene expression, the involvement of the PEA3 and AP-1 consensus sequences in amebic gene regulation was not clear from mutagenesis studies. URE4 is found upstream of at least one other *hgl* gene (55), and is bound by a nuclear factor (56). URE3, the only negative control element so far identified in *E. histolytica*, is also present in other

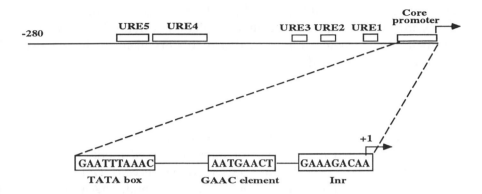

Figure 1. Regulatory elements at the *hgl5* promoter. Upstream regulatory elements and core promoter elements controlling the start of transcription at +1 are indicated. URE1, 2, 4 and 5 are positive elements, and URE3 is negative.

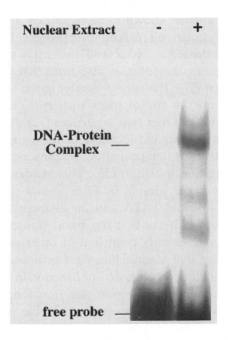

Figure 2. The URE3 element at the *hgl5* promoter is bound by nuclear protein. Electrophoretic mobility shift assay of (32) P-labelled double-stranded oligonucleotide corresponding to the URE3 element at the *hgl5* promoter was performed with nuclear extract from *E. histolytica* (46).

amebic genes (21, 51). URE3 is bound by a factor present in nuclear extracts (Fig. 2), and confers a growth-sensitive regulation of transcription on genes (46). As in other systems, it appears that regulatory elements lie upstream of a core promoter that determines the site of transcription initiation.

The Core Promoter

Comparison of the 5' flanking regions from 37 protein-coding genes of *E. histolytica* indicated the presence of three conserved motifs in the core promoter region (51). One of the three conserved sequences, (GTATTTAAAG/C), lies at −30 from the transcription start, the second, (AAAAATTCA), overlies the transcription start , and the third element, (GAAC), lies at variable locations between the first two sequences. These regions of the *hgl5* promoter were further defined by detailed mutational analysis of reporter constructs in transient and stable transfections (51, 52) (Fig. 1). The region at −30 (TATA box) was shown by positional analysis to control the site of transcription initiation (52) and has been shown to be bound by a factor in *E. histolytica* nuclear extracts (4). A putative TATA binding protein (TBP) has been reported for *E. histolytica* (GenBank Acc. No. Z48307) which is significantly divergent from the TBP of higher eukaryotes, as also from that of a fellow protozoan, *Plasmodium falciparum* (57). The region overlying the transcription initiation site (*Inr*) also controls the site of transcription initiation, but appears to play a lesser role than the other two sequences (52). A new third conserved element (GAAC), with variable location in the core promoter, has been shown to be important for determination of transcription start site and for efficiency of transcription initiation (58). This sequence is also specifically bound by a nuclear factor present in *E. histolytica* (58).

The presence of unusual TATA and *Inr* elements, and the presence of a novel third element indicate that the basal transcription machinery of *E. histolytica* differs significantly from that of other eukaryotes. This is not surprising considering that mammalian viral promoters do not function in *E. histolytica*, and amebic promoters do not function in mammalian cells (20). Study of the unique amebic core promoter function could identify novel transcription factors involved in aspects of amebic pathogenesis.

Pathogenicity and Signal Transduction

E. histolytica was named by Schaudinn in 1903 for its ability to destroy human tissues. Following colonisation of the colon, the parasite is able to penetrate through the mucin layer covering the colonic epithelium and thereby initiate the invasive process. The process of invasion is facilitated by the expression of virulence factors, a few of which have been identified and characterised. Several cysteine proteases and metalloproteinases are known to be secreted by trophozoites (59–62). Secretion of electron-dense granules (EDGs), whose contents include collagenases and gelatinases, appear to be associated with virulence in amebic trophozoites (24, 63, 64); antigens present in EDGs are detected mainly in virulent strains of *E. histolytica*, and a strain of *E. histolytica* that is mutant in cytoskeletal architecture and has reduced virulence, also has reduced EDG secretion. The presence of certain gram-negative bacteria has also been shown to enhance virulent functions of the trophozoite; adherence of bacteria to amebic trophozoites using either bacterial mannose-binding lectins or the amebic Gal/GalNAc lectin is able to increase the ameba-mediated lysis of cells in a tissue culture monolayer (65).

Destruction of the extracellular matrix, and cytolysis of host tissue are important aspects of invasion. Invasion of tissues requires also that the parasite adapt to an aerobic environment in comparison to the anaerobic colon, and that the parasite resist the host's immune response. Bacterial and red blood cell phagocytosis, and detoxification of heme are potentially important capabilities for the survival of the parasite within the host.

The involvement of signaling pathways in various aspects of pathogenesis of amebiasis is suggested from several studies (66), and they highlight the importance of the cytoskeleton in pathogenic functions of the trophozoite. The trophozoite undergoes cytoskeletal rearrangements in response to external signals, including interaction with erythrocytes and extracellular matrix (45, 61, 66, 67). Interaction with fibronectin has been shown to induce the release of proteases (61); an early response to fibronectin binding is the formation of actin adherence plates and focal contacts in trophozoites (61, 68) mediated by a Ca^{2+} influx (68) and activation of a protein kinase C signaling pathway (69). Phorbol esters that activate protein kinase C also specifically increase cytolytic activity of *E. histolytica*; sphingosine, a specific inhibitor of protein kinase C, inhibits cytolysis (70). Thus, different aspects of pathogenicity appear to rely on common signaling pathways.

Interaction with another extracellular matrix component, collagen, is believed to be mediated by an integrin-like receptor and induces secretion of collagenase-containing EDGs (24); Interaction with collagen also activates a signaling pathway involving phosphorylation of a focal adhesion kinase (pp125 FAK) and a mitogen induced protein kinase (MAPK) (71). Ca^{2+} and its specific binding protein calmodulin have been implicated in secretion of EDGs (72). A second Ca^{2+}-binding protein related to calmodulin has also been identified (73). Both of these Ca^{2+}-binding proteins have been shown to associate with Ca^{2+}-dependent protein kinases (74). Thus Ca^{2+}-dependent signaling plays an important role in *E. histolytica* pathogenesis.

Phagocytosis of bacteria and erythrocytes appears to involve signaling through p21^{rac} and phosphoinositide 3-kinase molecules (75). Genes for other components of signaling pathways that have been identified in *E. histolytica*, include *rho* and *rac* (76, 77) GTPases that are involved in numerous cellular functions, a *cdc2* protein kinase (9) that is involved in regulation of the cell-division cycle, and a *rac* protein serine/threonine kinase (78) that is also involved in multiple cellular processes. The non-pathogenic *E. dispar* strains appear to express lower levels of the *rac1* protein kinase RNA than *E. histolytica* (78).

The Gal/GalNAc lectin has been implicated in signal transduction events following adherence to host cell receptors (see below). Signaling pathways have also been implicated in the development of resistance to complement (see below).

Cytolysis

The cytolysis of host tissue is initiated following adherence of trophozoites to target cells. Adherence is mediated by a cell surface lectin; this lectin has also been implicated in the subsequent contact-dependent cell killing (79). This lectin is specific for galactose (Gal)/N-Acetyl-D-galactosamine (GalNAc), and both adherence and cytolysis are inhibitable by these sugars (79). Signal transduction events linked to adherence by the Gal/GalNAc lectin are thought to trigger the cytolytic response (see below). A second protein on the amebic cell-surface mediating interaction with Caco-2 cells has been reported that cross-reacts with CD44 antibody and has hyaluronic acid specificity (80); however, its role in pathogenicity of *E. histolytica* remains to be determined.

In vitro, trophozoites of *E. histolytica* will cause lysis of a wide range of tissue culture cell lines in addition to human neutrophils, T lymphocytes, and macrophages. The cytolytic activity of *E. histolytica* is contact dependent and extracellular (79). The steps involved in cytolysis have been extensively studied in vitro. In a matter of seconds following direct contact with an amebic trophozoite, intracellular calcium levels in the target cell rise about 20-fold, and are associated with membrane blebbing (81). Cell death is rapid, and occurs within 5–15 minutes. The acid pH of endocytic vesicles is important for the cytolytic event (82). The mechanism of target cell death may depend on the target cell type. Murine myeloid cells killed by amebic trophozoites undergo a Bcl2-independent apoptotic fragmentation of their DNA (83), while necrosis appears to predominate in human myeloid cells (84).

Pathogenic Factors

As indicated above, several factors contribute to the pathogenicity of *E. histolytica*, and some may yet be unidentified. However, three pathogenic factors have been extensively studied and characterised at the molecular level: the Gal/GalNAc lectin, mediating adherence to host cells, the amebapores that form pores in host cell membranes, and the cysteine proteinases that are cytopathic for host tissue.

The Gal/GalNAc Lectin in Adherence and Cytolysis

The surface borne lectin mediates adherence of the trophozoite to human colonic glycoproteins (85), human colonic epithelium (86), human neutrophils and erythrocytes (79, 87–89), a variety of cell culture lines (89–91), and to certain bacteria (64, 92). Mucins are highly polyvalent in terminal Gal and GalNAc residues, and synthetic polyvalent GalNAc glycoconjugates are bound by the lectin with very high affinity (93). Binding to colonic mucins appears to be a dynamic process, with trophozoites both degrading, and inducing the secretion of fresh mucins (85, 94). The human colonic mucin layer may be the first natural target for binding by trophozoites in the colon. The mucin layer may protect the host from contact-dependent cytolysis by neutralizing the binding epitopes on the lectin, while simultaneously providing a site of attachment for the colonizing parasite. Penetration through the mucin layer permits the trophozoite to invade and attack host tissue. The Gal/GalNAc lectin is also important in the cytolytic function following adherence: addition of Gal/GalNAc can inhibit cytolysis of target cells adhered to amebic trophozoites (87, 95). Different monoclonal antibodies to the lectin affect adherence and cytotoxicity functions differently, indicating that the lectin plays different functional roles (96). The related avirulent *E. dispar* also expresses a similar lectin on its surface; however, there are differences in epitope specificity (97), and the levels of GalNAc-inhibitable adherence appear to be lower (98).

Biochemistry

The carbohydrate determinants on host receptors for the Gal/GalNAc lectin have been defined using glycosylation mutants of the Chinese hamster ovary (CHO) cell line as targets for *E. histolytica* trophozoites (90, 91, 99). These studies showed that the Gal/GalNAc lectin mediates adherence to terminal N- and O- linked GalNAc and Gal residues on host cells. These residues are recognized by the lectin both when they are carried on glycoproteins or on glycosphingolipid glycans in liposomes (100, 101).

The purified Gal/GalNAc lectin was shown to be a 260 kDa heterodimer of heavy (170 kDa) and light (31/35 kDa) subunits linked by disulfide bonds (35, 102). Multiple genes encoding the heavy subunit have been sequenced (27, 28, 103). Using pulsed field gel electrophoresis, the heavy subunit was shown to be encoded by a family of 5 genes (*hgl1-5*) at 5 distinct loci (104) (Fig. 3). The basic organization of the gene family appears to be conserved in different isolates of *E. histolytica*. The *hgl* gene products are 89–95% identical at the amino-acid level and appear to be expressed at different levels as determined by RT-PCR of RNA derived from HM-1 : IMSS trophozoites grown in culture and from abscesses (104).

The heavy 170 kDa subunit has an amino-terminal hydrophobic signal sequence, a large extracellular domain containing 9 (*hgl2* product) or 16 (*hgl1* and *hgl3* products) potential sites of N-linked glycosylation, and a single putative transmembrane domain followed by a short cytoplasmic tail of 41 amino-acid residues (27, 28, 103). The protein is glycosylated; tunicamycin treatment blocked the glycosylation, and also blocked adherence (27). The protein also has domains that are cysteine-rich, and disulfide bonds appear to fold the protein into a protease-resistant structure (27). The lectin has been shown to cross-react with a monoclonal antibody to $\beta2$ integrins (105); the extracellular lectin sequence shares no significant amino-acid homology to integrins, and so the epitope similarity must be conformational.

Monoclonal antibodies that block or enhance adherence map to epitopes on the heavy subunit (106). However, the amino-acid sequences of the *hgl* or *lgl* gene products do not possess classical carbohydrate-binding motifs found in typical lectins, suggesting that the binding-sites may be unique (107, 108). In addition, antibodies to epitopes on the heavy subunit also block cytolysis (106). The adherence and cytolysis functions of the lectin appear to involve separate conformations of the molecule based on the differential effects of monoclonal antibodies on these functions (96).

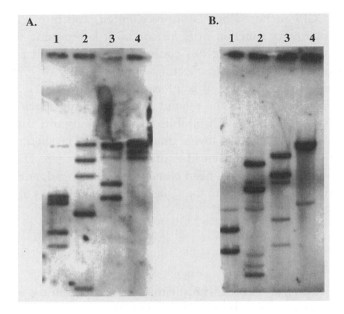

Figure 3. The Gal/GalNAc lectin is encoded by gene families. DNA from strain HM1 : IMSS was analyzed by clamped homogeneous electric field (CHEF) gel electrophoresis following digestion with restriction enzymes: 1, *EcoRV*; 2, *Hind*III; 3, *Xba*I; 4, *Xho*I. Duplicate sets of digests were hybridized in-gel with (32)-P labelled fragments of A. *hgl* and B. *lgl* genes and subjected to autoradiography. (With kind permission from Molecular Microbiology, Blackwell Science Ltd.), (104).

The light subunit (31/35 kDa) is encoded by a family of 6–7 *lgl* genes (36, 104, 109, 110). The *lgl* gene product has an amino-terminal signal peptide, and an unusually short 7 amino acid carboxyterminal glycosyl-phosphatidylinositol (GPI) anchor addition motif (36, 109, 110). The different *lgl* genes share 79–85% identity of sequence, and several of them are expressed in trophozoites (104). The light subunit has been shown to possess several isoforms (35, 36, 111). The 31 and 35 kDa isoforms have nearly identical amino acid compositions and CNBr-fragmentation patterns (35, 36). The 35 kDa form is more highly glycosylated and lacks the GPI anchor present on the 31 kDa form (36). The significance of the different isoforms is not presently clear.

The heavy and light subunits are only found in association with each other; heterodimerization may therefore be essential for stability of the lectin (111). The structure of the lectin with one membrane-spanning subunit, and a second GPI-anchored one is unprecedented, and implies that novel biochemical pathways function in *E. histolytica*. It is tempting to speculate that the presence of multiple genes coding for each subunit provides for variant forms of the heterodimeric lectin, with potentially diverse functions and capabilities. In this context, it is interesting to compare the lectin genes in *E. histolytica* with those of the related non-pathogenic species, *E. dispar*. *E. dispar* has Gal/GalNAc inhibitable adherence, ligand binding, and cytotoxicity functions that are lower than those of *E. histolytica* (98). Two *hgl* and four *lgl* genes have been identified in *E. dispar* (98, 112). The *hgl2* and *lgl1* genes of *E. dispar* have been cloned and sequenced, and show 86% and 80% identity, respectively, to the *E. histolytica* homologues at the amino-acid level (98, 112).

Cell signaling

The heterodimeric lectin is implicated in cell signaling in addition to adherence. Intracellular actin polymerization occurs at the contact interface of amebic trophozoites with Gal-terminal glycolipid liposomes (100); the negatively charged phospholipid was shown to be important for the actin polymerization (101). Colonic mucins bound by the lectin are rapidly endocytosed (94), and capped lectin has been shown to be directed to the uroid (113). Monoclonal antibodies to the lectin epitope 1 increase adherence but inhibit cytotoxicity (96, 106). Transfer of the lectin from trophozoites to epithelial monolayers following contact has been observed (114). In addition, the lectin has been implicated in amebic resistance to human complement (see below). All of these observations suggest that the lectin is involved in cell signaling events; a conformational change following adherence may precede downstream events. The cytoplasmic tail of the heavy subunit has several potential phosphorylation sites and is the most likely candidate for signal transduction (27, 28, 103) (Fig. 4). The possible involvement of the GPI-anchored light subunit in signal transduction cannot be ruled out, however, as there are examples of GPI-anchored proteins that transduce signals through interaction with transmembrane proteins (115).

Amoebapores

Amoebapores are a family of small proteins contained in cytoplasmic granules in the trophozoite; trophozoites are able to depolarize target cells

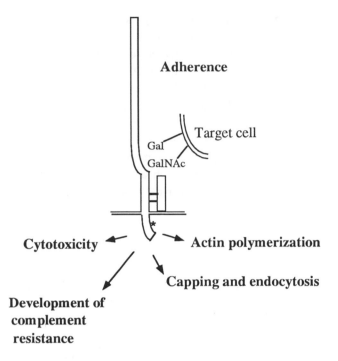

Figure 4. Model for the involvement of the Gal/GalNAc lectin in signal transduction. Following adherence, the cytoplasmic tail of the lectin is proposed to initiate (indicated by asterisk) multiple signalling events within the cell.

by the insertion of these pore-forming proteins that form ion-channels in their lipid membranes (116–119).

Three amoebapore isoforms of 77 amino acid residues, A, B, and C, have been characterized; these proteins have 35–57% sequence identity and are encoded by a family of three genes (30, 119). Amoebapores share significant homology with NK-lysins, which are pore-forming proteins present in natural killer (NK) cells and porcine cytotoxic T cells (120, 121), and they appear to have similar activities. Based on structure predictions and with the use of a genetic algorithm, the amoebapore structure has been modeled as a four amphipathic α-helix bundle, stabilized by disulfide bonds, a structure also conserved in NK-lysins (30, 122).

The three amebapore isoforms form ion-channels within lipid vesicles with varying kinetics (119). In addition to eukaryotic cell targets, amoebapores are effective in forming pores in bacterial membranes (119, 123). This antibacterial activity, directed at phagocytosed bacteria, has been proposed to be a primary function of amoebapores (124).

The non-pathogenic *E. dispar* trophozoites also contain amoebapores, but of lower activity (125). The amoebapore A of *E. dispar* is 95% identical to that from *E. histolytica*; one of the changes would result in a shortening of the putative amino-terminal α-helix of the *E. dispar* porin, and may contribute to lowered efficacy of amebapore function (125).

Amoebapores are not constitutively secreted by trophozoites into growth media (126). It has been proposed that amoebapores may be released to the outside of the cell upon stimulus, such as target cell contact, and thereby play a role in lysis of host cells during tissue invasion (124).

Cysteine Proteinases

E. histolytica trophozoites exhibit strong proteolytic activity and secrete copious amounts of cysteine proteinases into the growth media (22, 25, 127). Cysteine proteinases are constitutively released into the extracellular milieu by trophozoites in contrast to the regulated release of amoebapores (126).

Three isoforms of cysteine proteinases are produced in *E. histolytica* under conditions of growth in the laboratory (128). These proteins, of about 30 kDa, belong to the papain superfamily, and are encoded by three of a family of six genes (128–130). The non-pathogenic *E. dispar* trophozoites have four cysteine proteinase genes, but apparently only two of them are expressed (128). This could account for the overall low levels of cysteine proteinases expressed in *E. dispar*.

Cysteine proteinases have been implicated in the cytopathic effect of *E. histolytica* upon target cells, resulting in the release of adherent cells from monolayers, presumably by degradation of the anchoring proteins such as fibronectin and laminin (22, 25, 131). Consistent with the proposed cytopathogenic role, the administration of exogenous laminin or cysteine-proteinase inhibitor E-64 to neutralize cysteine proteinases was shown to greatly reduce the formation of amebic liver abscess in a severe combined immunodeficient (SCID) mouse model (132, 133).

Cysteine proteinases have also been shown to activate the alternate complement pathway by cleavage of C3 (134, 135). Anaphylatoxin products of complement cleavage, C3a and C5a, are degraded by the cysteine proteinases, thereby reducing the inflammatory response to infection (136). Serum and secretory IgA have been shown to be degraded by extracellular cysteine proteinases (137).

Complement Resistance

Invasion of the colon and dissemination through the blood stream exposes the parasite to the human complement system. Parasites isolated from invasive lesions show a high level of serum resistance; this complement resistance can be acquired in vitro by gradual exposure of trophozoites to increasing levels of non-immune serum (138–140). Trypsin-sensitive surface components are thought to confer complement-resistance, and this resistance was shown to be reversible (141, 142).

Virulent *E. histolytica* isolated from patients with invasive amebiasis activate the alternative complement pathway, but are resistant to C5b-9 complexes deposited on the membrane surface (134, 143). A monoclonal antibody to the heavy subunit epitopes 6 and 7 of the Gal/GalNAc lectin increases amebic lysis by human serum, and by purified complement components C5b-9 (144). The sequence of the heavy subunit shows limited homology to CD59, a human inhibitor of C5b-9 assembly, and the purified lectin is recognized by anti-CD59 antibodies. The lectin binds purified C8 and C9 components, and prevents assembly of the membrane-attack complex on the amebic membrane. Lectin purified from serum-resistant amebae was able to confer C5b-9 resistance to serum-sensitive amebae, directly demonstrating its C5b-9 inhibitory activity (144). This raises the possibility that there are lectin isoforms that are able to confer different complement resistance phenotypes.

Subtractive cDNA library screening of complement-resistant and sensitive amebae has been carried out to identify genes that are expressed at elevated levels in complement-resistant amebae; a putative serine/threonine kinase was identified in this screen (7), suggesting the involvement of a signaling cascade in the acquisition or maintenance of complement resistance.

Future Prospects

Recent advances in the molecular biology of *E. histolytica* have made it possible to better understand the organism and the factors contributing to its pathogenicity. It has provided the ability to characterize the mechanisms of immunity, and potentiated the development of candidate vaccines. The cloning and analysis of multiple genes has made it clear that the *E. histolytica* genes are different in many ways from their counterparts in higher eukaryotes, and from other protozoans. This information may help to pinpoint targets for development of new drug therapy in the future.

PCR techniques have now made it possible to identify isolates of *E. histolytica* (145); this will provide the tools for epidemiological studies worldwide. It potentially will also permit correlation of pathogenicity with expression of particular genes.

The ability to transfect the organism, both transiently (19–21) and stably (53, 54), with foreign DNA has opened the door to manipulation of its genome. The study of transcription mechanisms is underway in several laboratories, and a wealth of information regarding regulation of transcription at various

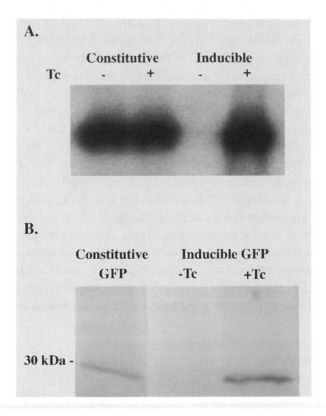

Figure 5. Tetracycline-inducible expression (148) of RNA and protein in *E. histolytica* trophozoites. A. Northern blot analysis of RNA from trophozoites expressing the luciferase gene under control of a constitutive or inducible *hgl5* promoter and probed with a luciferase gene fragment. B. Western blot analysis of lysates from trophozoites expressing the GFP protein under control of a constitutive or inducible *hgl5* promoter using GFP-specific antiserum as primary antibody.

promoters should soon be available. Functional analysis of gene products has also been advanced. For instance, over- expression of the P-glycoprotein1 has been shown to confer a multidrug resistance phenotype (146). The involvement of signal transduction intermediates in phagocytosis has also been demonstrated (75). The applicability of antisense RNA technology to amebic gene expression can be fully explored. With the recent development of inducible expression systems (147, 148), it is now possible to express gene products in amebic trophozoites in a controlled manner (Fig. 5). The ability to regulate the expression of mutant and potentially toxic gene products should permit the detailed functional analysis of genes contributing to the pathogenicity of *E. histolytica*.

Current efforts directed at developing techniques for further genetic manipulation of the parasite, such as integration of foreign DNA in the genome and gene knockouts, will provide new insights into aspects of chromosome structure and ploidy, and a better handle on the funtional analysis of pathogenic factors in *E. histolytica*.

Acknowledgements

The work carried out in the author's laboratory is supported by grant AI37941 from the National Institutes of Health. We acknowledge our colleagues in the field of amebiasis who have been responsible for the rapid advances in our understanding of *E. histolytica*. The literature in the field is voluminous, and we apologize for any inadvertent omissions in the citation of relevant literature.

Note Added in Proof

In the several months following submission of this chapter, many few findings regarding the molecular and cellular characterization of *E. histolytica* have been reported. We regret that we cannot now include them all, but would like to cite ones with special relevance to this review. A linkage map has been established for the *E. histolytica* genome with 14 linkage groups and a likely ploidy of 4 (149). With regard to the pathogenic factors, a membrane-bound cysteine proteinase specific for *E. histolytica* and lacking in *E. dispar* has been characterized (150). A Gal/GalNAc ligand binding domain has been located on the extracellular portion of the Hgl subunit of the Gal/GalNAc lectin (151, 152). Several new approaches to genetic manipulation of the amebic genome have been initiated: inducible expression of dominant-negative mutants of the Gal/GalNAc lection (153), successful inhibition of cysteine proteinases and the Gal/GalNAc lectin light subunit by expression of antisense RNA (154–156) and retroviral integration in the genomic DNA (!57).

References

1. Gelderman AH, *et al.* (1971). *J. Parasitol.* **57**: 912.
2. Char S and Farthing MJG (1992). *Int. J. Protozool.* **22**: 381.
3. Tannich E and Horstmann RD (1992). *J. Mol. Evol.* **34**: 272.
4. Bruchhaus I, *et al.* (1993). *DNA Cell. Biol.* **12**: 925.
5. Gangopadhyay SS, *et al.* (1997). *Mol. Biochem. Parasitol.* **89**: 73.
6. De Meester F, *et al.* (1991). *Mol. Biochem. Parasitol.* **44**: 23.
7. Urban B, *et al.* (1996). *Mol. Biochem. Parasitol.* **80**: 171.
8. Ramos MA, *et al.* (1997). *Mol. Biochem. Parasitol.* **88**: 225.
9. Lohia A and Samuelson J (1993). *Gene* **127**: 203.
10. Plaimauer B, *et al.* (1993). *DNA Cell Biol.* **12**: 89.
11. Miranda R, *et al.* (1996). *Gene* **180**: 37.
12. Lioutas C and Tannich E (1995). *Mol. Biochem. Parasitol.* **73**: 259.
13. Quon DVK, *et al.* (1996). *J. Mol. Evol.* **43**: 253.
14. Bhattacharya S, *et al.* (1989). *J. Protozool.* **36**: 455.
15. Huber JB, *et al.* (1989). *Mol. Biochem. Parasitol.* **32**: 285.
16. Sehgal D, *et al.* (1994). *Mol. Biochem. Parasitol.* **67**: 205.
17. Mittal V, *et al.* (1991). *Nuc. Acids Res.* **19**: 2777.
18. Dhar SK, *et al.* (1996). *Mol. Cell Biol.* **16**: 2314.
19. Nickel R and Tannich E (1994). *Proc. Natl. Acad. Sci. USA* **91**: 7095.
20. Purdy JE, *et al.* (1994). *Proc. Natl. Acad. Sci. USA* **91**: 7099.
21. Gilchrist CA, *et al.* (1995). *Mol. Biochem. Parasitol.* **74**: 1.
22. Lushbaugh WB, *et al.* (1984). *Gastroenterology* **87**: 17.
23. Agrawal A, *et al.* (1989). *J. Protozool.* **36**: 90.
24. Munoz ML, *et al.* (1990). *J. Clin. Microbiol.* **28**: 2418.
25. Keene WE, *et al.* (1990). *Exp. Parasitol.* **71**: 199.
26. Stanley SL, *et al.* (1990). *Proc. Natl. Acad. Sci. USA* **87**: 4976.
27. Mann BJ, *et al.* (1991). *Proc. Natl. Acad. Sci. USA* **88**: 3248.
28. Tannich E, *et al.* (1991). *Proc. Natl. Acad. Sci. USA* **88**: 1849.
29. Tannich E, *et al.* (1992). *Mol. Biochem. Parasitol.* **54**: 109.

30. Leippe M, *et al.* (1992). *EMBO J.* **11**: 3501.
31. Zhang W-W, *et al.* (1994). *Mol. Biochem. Parasitol.* **63**: 157.
32. Yang W, *et al.* (1994). *Mol. Biochem. Parasitol.* **64**: 253.
33. Stanley SL, *et al.* (1995). *J. Biol. Chem.* **270**: 4121.
34. de la Vega H, *et al.* (1997). *Mol. Biochem. Parasitol.* **85**: 139.
35. Petri Jr. WA, *et al.* (1989). *J. Biol. Chem.* **264**: 3007.
36. McCoy JJ, *et al.* (1993). *J. Biol. Chem.* **268**: 24223.
37. Diamond LS, *et al.* (1974) *Arch. Invest. Med.* **5**: 423.
38. Das SR and Goshal S (1976). *Ann. Trop. Med. Parasitol.* **70**: 439.
39. Lushbaugh WB, *et al.* (1978). *Am. J. Trop. Med. Hyg.* **27**: 248.
40. Meerovitch E and Ghadirian E (1978). *Arch. Invest. Med.* **9 (Suppl I)**: 253.
41. Wittner M and Rosenbaum RM (1970). *Am. J. Trop. Med. Hyg.* **19**: 755.
42. Bracha R and Mirelman D (1984). *J. Exp. Med.* **160**: 353.
43. Brucchaus I and Tannich E (1994). *Mol. Biochem. Parasitol.* **67**: 281.
44. Flores BM, *et al.* (1996). *J. Inf. Dis.* **173**: 226.
45. Manning-Cela R and Meza I (1997). *J. Euk. Microbiol.* **44**: 18.
46. Gilchrist CA, *et al.* (1996). *Inf. Immun.* **66**: 2383.
47. Descoteaux S, *et al.* (1995). *Gene* **164**: 179.
48. Sanchez LB, *et al.* (1994). *Mol. Biochem. Parasitol.* **67**: 125.
49. Sanchez LB, *et al.* (1994). *Mol. Biochem. Parasitol.* **67**: 137.
50. Buβ H, *et al.* (1995). *Mol. Biochem. Parasitol.* **72**: 1.
51. Purdy JE, *et al.* (1996). *Mol. Biochem. Parasitol.* **78**: 91.
52. Singh U, *et al.* (1997). *Proc. Natl. Acad. Sci. USA* **94**: 8812.
53. Hamann L, *et al.* (1995). *Proc. Natl. Acad. Sci. USA* **92**: 8975.
54. Vines RR, *et al.* (1995). *Mol. Biochem. Parasitol.* **71**: 265.
55. Purdy JE (1996). Ph.D. Dissertation, Univ. of Virginia.
56. Schaenman JM, *et al.* (1998). *Mol. Biochem. Parasitol.* **94**: 309.
57. McAndrew MB, *et al.* (1993). *Gene* **124**: 165.
58. Singh U and Rogers JB (1998). *J. Biol. Chem.* **273**: 21663.
59. Lushbaugh W, *et al.* (1985). *Exp. Parasitol.* **59**: 328.
60. Munoz ML, *et al.* (1982). *J. Exp. Med.* **155**: 42.
61. Talamas-Rohana P and Meza I (1988). *J. Cell Biol.* **106**: 1787.
62. Que X and Reed SL (1997). *Parasitol. Today* **13**: 190.
63. Serrano JJ, *et al.* (1994). *Mol. Microbiol.* **11**: 787.
64. Leon G, *et al.* (1997). *Mol. Biochem. Parasitol.* **85**: 233.
65. Bracha R and Mirelman D (1984). *J. Exp. Med.* **160**: 353.
66. Guillen N (1996). *Trends Microbiol.* **4**: 191.
67. Bailey GB, *et al.* (1985). *J. Exp. Med.* **162**: 546.

68. Carbajal ME, *et al.* (1996). *Exp. Parasitol.* **82**: 11.
69. Santiago A, *et al.* (1994). *Exp. Parasitol.* **79**: 436.
70. Weikel C, *et al.* (1988). *Inf. Immun.* **56**: 1485.
71. Perez E, *et al.* (1996). *Exp. Parasitol.* **82**: 164.
72. Munoz ML, *et al.* (1991). *Mol. Microbiol.* **5**: 1707.
73. Prasad J, *et al.* (1992). *Mol. Biochem. Parasitol.* **52**: 137.
74. Yadava N, *et al.* (1997). *Mol. Biochem. Parasitol.* **84**: 69.
75. Ghosh SK and Samuelson J (1997). *Inf. Immun.* **65**: 4243.
76. Lohia A and Samuelson J (1993). *Mol. Biochem. Parasitol.* **58**: 177.
77. Lohia A and Samuelson J (1996). *Gene* **173**: 205.
78. Que X, *et al.* (1993). *Mol. Biochem. Parasitol.* **60**: 161.
79. Ravdin JI and Guerrant RL (1981). *J. Clin. Invest.* **68**: 1305.
80. Renesto P, *et al.* (1997). *Inf. Immun.* **65**: 4330.
81. Ravdin JI, *et al.* (1988). *Inf. Immun.* **56**: 1505.
82. Ravdin JI, *et al.* (1986). *J. Protozool.* **33**: 478.
83. Ragland BD, *et al.* (1994). *Exp. Parasitol.* **79**: 460.
84. Berninghausen O and Leippe M (1997). *Inf. Immun.* **65**: 3615.
85. Chadee K, *et al.* (1987). *J. Clin. Invest.* **80**: 1245.
86. Ravdin JI, *et al.* (1985). *Inf. Immun.* **48**: 292.
87. Guerrant RL, *et al.* (1981). *J. Inf. Dis.* **143**: 83.
88. Burchard GD, *et al.* (1992). *Parasitol. Res.* **78**: 336.
89. Burchard GD and Bilke R (1992). *Parasitol. Res.* **78**: 146.
90. Li E, *et al.* (1988). *J. Exp. Med.* **167**: 1725.
91. Li E, *et al.* (1989). *Inf. Immun.* **57**: 8.
92. Bracha R and Mirelman D (1983). *Inf. Immun.* **40**: 882.
93. Adler P, *et al.* (1995). *J. Biol. Chem.* **270**: 5164.
94. Chadee K, *et al.* (1988). *J. Infect. Dis.* **158**: 398.
95. Ravdin JI, *et al.* (1980). *J. Exp. Med.* **152**: 377.
96. Petri Jr WA, *et al.* (1990). *J. Immunol.* **144**: 4803.
97. Petri Jr WA, *et al.* (1990). *Inf. Immun.* **58**: 1802.
98. Dodson JM, *et al.* (1997). *Parasitol. International.*
99. Ravdin JI, *et al.* (1989). *Inf. Immun.* **57**: 2179.
100. Bailey GB, *et al.* (1990). *Inf. Immun.* **58**: 43.
101. Bailey GB, *et al.* (1990). *Inf. Immun.* **58**: 2389.
102. Petri Jr WA, *et al.* (1987). *J. Clin. Invest.* **80**: 1238.
103. Purdy JE, *et al.* (1993). *Mol. Biochem. Parasitol.* **62**: 53.
104. Ramakrishnan G, *et al.* (1996). *Mol. Microbiol.* **19**: 91.
105. Adams SA, *et al.* (1993). *The Lancet* **341**: 17.
106. Mann BJ, *et al.* (1993). *Inf. Immun.* **61**: 1772.

107. Rini JM (1995). *Ann. Rev. Biophys. Biomol. Struct.* **24**: 551.
108. Barondes SH, *et al.* (1994). *J. Biol. Chem.* **269**: 20807.
109. McCoy JJ, *et al.* (1993). *Mol. Biochem. Parasitol.* **61**: 325.
110. Tannich E, *et al.* (1992). *Mol. Biochem. Parasitol.* **55**: 225.
111. McCoy JJ, *et al.* (1994). *Glycoconj. J.* **11**: 432.
112. Pillai DR, *et al.* (1997). *Mol. Biochem. Parasitol.* **87**: 101.
113. Arhets P, *et al.* (1995). *Inf. Immun.* **63**: 4358.
114. Leroy A, *et al.* (1995). *Inf. Immun.* **63**: 4253.
115. Sitrin RG, *et al.* (1996). *J. Clin. Invest.* **97**: 1942.
116. Lynch EC, *et al.* (1982). *EMBO J.* **801**.
117. Young JD-E, *et al.* (1982). *J. Exp. Med.* **156**: 1677.
118. Rosenberg I, *et al.* (1989). *Mol. Biochem. Parasitol.* **33**: 237.
119. Leippe M, *et al.* (1994). *Mol. Microbiol.* **14**: 895.
120. Andersson M, *et al.* (1995). *EMBO J.* **14**: 1615.
121. Leippe M (1995). *Cell* **83**: 17.
122. Dandekar T and Leippe M (1997). *Folding and Design* **2**: 47.
123. Leippe M, *et al.* (1994). *Proc. Natl. Acad. Sci. USA* **91**: 2602.
124. Leippe M (1997). *Parasitol. Today* **13**: 178.
125. Leippe M, *et al.* (1993). *Mol. Biochem. Parasitol.* **59**: 101.
126. Leippe M, *et al.* (1995). *Parasitol.* **111**: 569.
127. Luaces L and Barrett AJ (1988). *Biochem. J.* **250**: 903.
128. Brucchaus I, *et al.* (1996). *Mol. Microbiol.* **22**: 255.
129. Tannich E, *et al.* (1991). *Mol. Biochem. Parasitol.* **49**: 61.
130. Reed SL, *et al.* (1993). *J. Clin. Invest.* **91**: 1532.
131. Schulte W and Scholze HJ (1989). *Protozool.* **36**: 538.
132. Li E, *et al.* (1995). *Inf. Immun.* **63**: 4150.
133. Stanley SL, *et al.* (1995). *Inf. Immun.* **63**: 1587.
134. Reed SL, *et al.* (1986). *J. Immunol.* **136**: 2265.
135. Reed SL, *et al.* (1989). *J. Immunol.* **143**: 189.
136. Reed SL, *et al.* (1995). *J. Immunol.* **155**: 266.
137. Kelsall BL and Ravdin JI (1993). *J. Inf. Dis.* **168**: 1319.
138. Calderon J and Tovar R (1986). *Immunol.* **58**: 467.
139. Mogyoros M, *et al.* (1986). *Isr. J. Med. Sci.* **22**: 915.
140. Hamelmann C, *et al.* (1992). *Parasite Immunol.* **14**: 23.
141. Hamelmann C, *et al.* (1993). *Parasite Immunol.* **15**: 223.
142. Hamelmann C, *et al.* (1993). *Inf. Immun.* **61**: 1636.
143. Reed SL and Gigli I (1990). *J. Clin. Invest.* **86**: 1815.
144. Braga LL, *et al.* (1992). *J. Clin. Invest.* **90**: 1131.
145. Clark CG and Diamond LS (1993). *Exp. Parasitol.* **77**: 450.

146. Ghosh SK, *et al.* (1996). *Mol. Biochem. Parasitol.* **82**: 257.
147. Hamann L, *et al.* (1997). *Mol. Biochem. Parasitol.* **84**: 83.
148. Ramakrishnan G, *et al.* (1997). *Mol. Biochem. Parasitol.* **84**: 93.
149. Willhoeft U and Tannich E (1999). *Mol. Biochem. Parasitol.* **99**: 41.
150. Jacobs T, *et al.* (1998). *Mol. Microbiol.* **27**: 269.
151. Dodson JM, *et al.* (1999). *J. Inf. Dis.* **179**: 460.
152. Pillai DR, *et al.* (1999). *Inf. Immun.* **67**: 3836.
153. Vines RR, *et al.* (1998). *Mol. Biol. of the Cell* **9**: 2069.
154. Ankri S, *et al.* (1998). *Mol. Microbiol.* **28**: 777.
155. Ankri S, *et al.* (1999). *Inf. Immun.* **67**: 421.
156. Ankri S, *et al.* (1999). *Mol. Microbiol.* **33**: 327.
157. Que X, *et al.* (1999). *Mol. Biochem. Parasitol.* **99**: 237.

Chapter 5

Clinical Manifestations and Diagnosis

SL Reed

Departments of Pathology and Medicine
UCSD Medical Center, 200 W. Arbor Dr.
San Diego, Ca 92103-8416, USA
E-mail: slreed@ucsd.edu

An estimated 10% of the world's population is infected with *E. histolytica* and *E. dispar* with associated mortality rates that are second only to malaria and schistosomiasis (1). International travel and large immigrant populations have caused infection with *E. histolytica* to emerge as a problem in industrial nations as well. The diagnosis of intestinal and extraintestinal amebiasis can be challenging to western physicians as symptoms mimic many other diseases. Recent advances in our understanding of the pathogenesis of amebiasis however, have had a significant impact on the early diagnosis and treatment of amebic infection (Reviewed in (2–4)). Furthermore, separation of *Entamoeba* into *E. histolytica*, which can cause invasive disease, and *E. dispar*, which cannot, allows the clinician to focus on early identification and treatment of *E. histolytica* infection in the minority of patients who are at highest personal risk and pose a major public health problem.

Clinical Manifestations: Intestinal Amebiasis

Asymptomatic Colonization

Asymptomatic cyst passage is the most common manifestation of intestinal *Entamoeba* infection. Studies carried out before the separation of *E. histolytica* and *E. dispar* found that the majority of asymptomatic carriers spontaneously cleared their infection within five months (5). It is now appreciated that the majority of these patients, even in highly endemic areas, harbored *E. dispar* (previously referred to as nonpathogenic *E. histolytica* (6). Even patients with

AIDS who were infected with *E. dispar* resolved their infections successfully without histologic evidence of invasion (7–9), confirming the noninvasive genotype of *E. dispar*. It is important, however, to identify not only patients with frank amebiasis, but also the rare patient who is asymptomatically colonized with *E. histolytica* because they are a public health risk through the shedding of infectious cysts. Ten percent of asymptomatic patients infected with *E. histolytica* in South Africa developed colitis within one year (10), emphasising the importance to the colonised patients and their contacts of early diagnosis and treatment.

Amebic Colitis

Patients with amebic colitis usually note the gradual onset of abdominal pain and watery stools containing mucus and blood. In contrast to bacterial causes of dysentery, fever in early amebic colitis is uncommon, occurring in only one-third of patients (11). Eighty percent of patients complain of localised abdominal pain (11). Some patients may only have intermittent diarrhea alternating with constipation. If left untreated, a number of patients spontaneously resolve their symptoms.

The earliest pathologic changes in intestinal invasion have been documented in gerbils, hamsters (12–14) or in SCID mice with human intestinal xenografts (15). *E. histolytica* trophozoites cause thinning of the mucous layer followed by shortening of the microvilli even before attachment (14). Apical separation of the epithelial cells is mediated by the action of extracellular cysteine proteinases which degrade components of the extracellular matrix, including collagen, elastin, and laminin (16, 17). Trophozoites attach via the galactose-inhibitable lectin to mucus and epithelial cells (18, 19). Host cell lysis requires direct contact and is mediated by phospholipases (20), pore-forming proteins (21), and hemolysins (22). An influx of acute inflammatory cells follows early amebic invasion (12). The acute cellular infiltrate is initiated by release of chemoattractant and proinflammatory chemokines (IL-8, GROα, GM-CSF, IL-1α, and IL-6) by lysed host cells (23). Release of IL-8, a potent attractor and activator of neutrophils, can also be stimulated from epithelial cells by whole trophozoites or amebic proteins without direct cell contact (24). These *in vitro* findings were confirmed *in vivo* in human intestinal xenografts (15). Trophozoites erode through the lamina propria and extend laterally producing the characteristic flask-shaped ulcer (Fig. 1). At sigmoidoscopy, amebic colitis is characterized by eroded ulcers surrounded

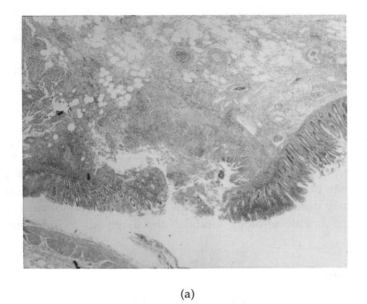

(a)

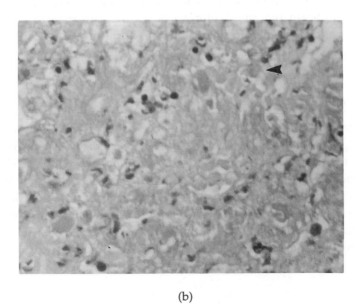

(b)

Figure 1. Pathology of amebic colitis. A. Flask-shaped ulcer with acute inflammatory cells and undermining of epithelium. B. Trophozoites marked with arrow (H&E stain, 400X).

by normal appearing epithelium. Microscopically, trophozoites are readily detected in the necrotic tissue by haematoxylin-eosin or periodic acid-Schiff staining.

Fulminant colitis, with severe bloody diarrhea, fever, and abdominal pain, is usually a pediatric disease (25). An unusual complication of intestinal infection, fulminant colitis progresses to colonic perforation in 60% of patients (26).

Fewer than 1% of patients with active intestinal infection develop a mass-like lesion or ameboma (11). If abdominal pain and mass lesions are found in the setting of dysentery, the diagnosis is made more easily. Some patients, however, may present with asymptomatic mass lesions. On barium enema, the lesion may mimic carcinoma, but the presence of trophozoites on biopsy or a positive amebic serology establish the diagnosis of ameboma.

Complications

The most serious complication of amebic colitis is perforation and secondary bacterial peritonitis, which may present acutely or subacutely (11). Perforation may also complicate toxic megacolon following inappropriate steroid therapy and present as diffuse colonic distension with intramural gas (27). Significant hemorrhage is unusual (11).

Differential Diagnosis

The major differential of acute amebic colitis is bacillary dysentery caused by *Shigella, Salmonella, Campylobacter, Yersinia,* or entero-invasive *E. coli.* Like amebiasis, all of these pathogens are associated with grossly bloody or heme positive stools. Significant leukocytes are less common in amebic infection than bacterial dysentery, and patients usually are afebrile. Amebic colitis can also be very difficult to differentiate from inflammatory bowel disease. Because of the potentially serious complications of steroid treatment in acute amebiasis, amebic infection must be ruled out by biopsy and serology before instituting therapy for inflammatory bowel disease (27).

Extraintestinal Amebiasis

Amebic liver abscess is the most common manifestation of extraintestinal disease. The clinical presentation is highly variable, ranging from obvious

Table 1. Presenting symptoms in patients with amebic liver abscess.

	DeBakey & Oschner (73)	Adams & MacLeod (35)	Katzenstein et al. (28)
Number of patients	263	2,074	67
Length of symptoms			
Acute (< 2 wks.)	—	59%	66%
Chronic (< 2 wks.)	—	41%	34%
Fever	87%	75%	67%
Abdominal pain	88%	62%	68%
Diarrhea	27%	14%	30%
Cough	—	11%	10%
Weight loss	53%	—	33%

infection of the liver, to prominent pulmonary symptoms, to fever of unknown origin. The cardinal manifestations are right upper quadrant pain and fever (Table 1). Pain may be local or referred to the right shoulder. Patients who present acutely with symptoms of less than two weeks duration, have more prominent abdominal pain with fevers and rigors (28).

Other patients present with a chronic illness lasting longer than two weeks. They tend to be older, have less fever (only 30%), and may have a wasting disease with significant weight loss (28). In more recent series, the number of patients presenting with acute disease may be increasing, possibly reflecting earlier diagnosis and better access to medical care (28).

Only a minority of patients (30%) have active dysentery at the time of presentation with an amebic liver abscess (28). However, daily stool cultures revealed that 72% harbored *E. histolytica* despite an absence of symptoms (29).

Trophozoites reach the liver through the portal venous system causing periportal inflammation. To survive dissemination through the bloodstream, *E. histolytica* trophozoites are resistant to the lytic action of complement (30, 31), a virulence property common to many pathogens causing disseminated infection (32, 33). Amebic hepatitis has been postulated, but there is no pathologic basis of the syndrome. Despite the same early influx of acute inflammatory cells seen in amebic colitis, *E. histolytica* trophozoites rapidly lyse inflammatory and host cells, causing rapid expansion of the abscess

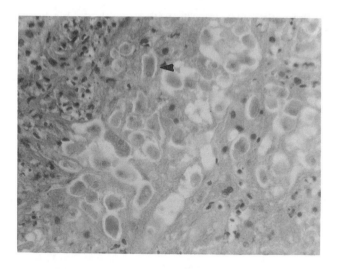

Figure 2. Pathology of amebic liver abscess. Biopsy of amebic liver abscess demonstrated necrosis with trophozoites (arrow) near capsule. (H&E stain, 400X).

filled with necrotic, proteinaceous debris. Trophozoites, if present, are only detectable in the edge of the abscess (Fig. 2).

Pulmonary symptoms may also be prominent; a nonproductive cough was noted by 80% of patients in some series (34). In as many as 15% of patients, fever is the only symptom, emphasising that the diagnosis of amebic liver abscess must be considered in the differential diagnosis of fever of unknown origin (28).

Fever is the most common physical finding, with a prevalence of 80% (Table 2). The majority of patients also have a tender liver, especially if they present acutely. Hepatomegaly is present in half, particularly if symptoms have been present for several weeks.

Complications

The most serious complications of amebic liver abscess are rupture, particularly into the pericardium, and superinfection. Rupture into the pleura is most common and usually has a good prognosis. Bacterial superinfection at initial presentation is very unusual, but the risk increases to 10% with repeated aspiration (35). With early diagnosis and therapy, the mortality of uncomplicated amebic liver abscess is less than 1% (35).

Table 2. Physical findings in patients with amebic liver abscess.

	DeBakey & Oschner (73)	Adams & MacLeod (35)	Katzenstein et al. (28)
Number of patients	263	2,074	67
Fever	87%	75%	90%
Tender liver	89%	80%	90%
Hepatomegaly	77%	—	43%
Rales/rhonchi	—	47%	43%
Jaundice	13%	—	10%

Pleuropulmonary Amebiasis

Thoracic involvement is the most common complication of an amebic liver abscess, occurring in up to 35% of patients (35, 36). Complaints usually include pleuritic chest pain, cough, and dyspnea. The four major patterns of pulmonary involvement are: (1) serous effusion, (2) consolidation or abscess formation, (3) empyema, and (4) hepatobronchial fistula (35). As many as 50% of patients develop serous pleural effusions which resolves spontaneously (37). Lung abscesses or consolidation occur in up to 10% of patients with amebic liver abscess. Radiographic findings may be slow to resolve, but medical therapy alone usually is sufficient (35, 38). Hepatobronchial fistulas may present dramatically with cough productive of necrotic liver, which may contain trophozoites (35, 38, 39). Before the advent of effective medical therapy, the development of an hepatobronchial fistula was considered a good prognostic sign because it rapidly decompressed the abscess.

Rupture of an abscess into the pleural space with empyema formation can cause sudden respiratory compromise (40, 41). Adequate drainage with medical therapy is key, but the mortality may still approach 15–30% (37, 41).

Peritoneal Amebiasis

Intraperitoneal rupture, with a prevalence of 2–7.5% of patients, is the second most common complication of amebic liver abscess (35, 42). Because the contents of amebic liver abscesses are sterile, intraperitoneal rupture is not as serious as colonic rupture with secondary bacterial peritonitis. Medical therapy and percutaneous drainage are the optimal treatment.

Pericardial Amebiasis

Rupture into the pericardium poses the greatest risk to patients with amebic liver abscess, with mortality rates approaching 70% in older series (43). With better imaging techniques, serous pericardial effusions may be recognized more frequently. Rupture into the pericardium may present as progressive tamponade or acute shock (35, 44). Pericardial rupture can occur even when patients are on medical therapy, which provides the rationale for recommending aspiration of all abscesses of the left lobe of the liver (45).

Cerebral Amebiasis

Cerebral amebiasis, usually detected only at autopsy, occured in 1–2% of patients who died prior to the advent of adequate medical therapy (46, 47). The symptoms, which depend on the size and location of the lesion(s), include headache, vomiting, vertigo, seizures, and abnormal mental status (46). The possibility of cerebral involvement should be considered in any patient with amebiasis and abnormal mental status. A number of cases have been successfully treated with medical therapy alone (48, 49), and the frequency of this complication will probably continue to decrease with the excellent CNS penetration of the nitroimidazoles.

Genitourinary Amebiasis

Renal involvement in amebiasis is very rare as no cases were detected in the largest clinical series (35). Extension from either an amebic liver abscess or retroperitoneal colonic perforation is the most likely etiology (50). Optimal therapy includes both aspiration and medical therapy (51).

Genital involvement occurs secondary to the development of fistuale from amebic liver abscesses or colitis or as primary infection by sexual transmission (52–54). Lesions usually present as painful, punched out ulcers which must be distinguished from carcinoma, tuberculosis, chancroid, and lymphogranuloma venereum (53, 54). Biopsy may show trophozoites and allow the diagnosis of a very treatable lesion (53, 54).

Differential Diagnosis of Amebic Liver Abscess

Diagnosis of amebic liver abscesses can be very challenging because of the wide range of presenting syndromes. The diagnosis should be considered in any patient with fever, symptoms referable to the right upper quadrant, or space-occupying lesions of the liver. The most frequent problem is to differentiate between amebic and pyogenic liver abscesses. The patient with a pyogenic abscess is usually more than 50 years old and quite ill, presenting with fever, pain, and a previous history of gastrointestinal tract disease (55). If a pyogenic abscess is a consideration, the abscess must be drained to establish the correct diagnosis and provide an essential element of the treatment pyogenic abscesses (45).

Diagnosis of Amebiasis

Chemistry and Hematology Testing

Abnormalities in routine laboratory testing are not specific for amebiasis. More than 75% of patients have an elevated total white blood cell count (28), particularly patients presenting with symptoms for less than ten days. As with other invasive protozoal diseases, eosinophilia is not a feature. If present, anemia is typically normochromic and normocytic.

The only consistent abnormality in blood chemistries is an elevated alkaline phosphatase, which is present in more than 75% of patients with amebic liver abscesses (28). Elevated transaminases are present only in patients who present acutely or with multiple abscesses (28).

Microscopic Diagnosis

The identification of hematophagous trophozoites is the hallmark of *E. histolytica* infection. Examination of a fresh stool or scrapings from an ulcer for motile trophozoites is optimal. Trophozoites are readily killed by water, barium, antibiotics, or dessication, so examination of trichrome-stained concentrates of three fresh stools is also important. In amebic liver abscesses, trophozoites are usually only present in the capsule and are rarely detected by aspiration. Culture is more sensitive than examination of trichrome stained slides, but is not routinely available. *E. histolytica* and *E. dispar* are morphologically identical and cannot be differentiated by microscopy alone without the presence of phagocytosed erythrocytes in *E. histolytica*. A recent WHO special committee recommended that quadrinucleate cysts now be identified as *E. histolytica/E. dispar* (56).

Identification of *E. histolytica* and *E. dispar*

A number of tests are now available to differentiate *E. histolytica* from *E. dispar*, including isoenzyme analysis, ELISA, and PCR. Isoenzyme analysis, developed by Sargeaunt (57) first allowed the separation of *E. histolytica* based on the distinct patterns of four enzymes or zymodemes. These studies of more than 3,000 clinical isolates provided the first reliable method of speciating *Entamoeba*. Isoenzyme analysis remains primarily a research technique, however, and requires primary amebic cultures. An ELISA-based assay differentiates between *E. histolytica* and *E. dispar* by taking advantage of the unique epitopes of the galactose-inhibitable lectin of *E. histolytica*. In extensive studies in Egypt, South Africa, and Bangladesh, the heavy subunit of the lectin can be detected in blood (58) and in feces with a sensitivity of 80% and a specificity of 99% (59). This ELISA-based assay for stool is now commercially available in the United States.

A number of PCR-based assays have been developed for direct detection of *E. histolytica* and *E. dispar* in stools. The species can be differentiated by amplification of the repetitive regions in extrachromosomal DNA (60, 61), small subunit rRNA (62), or the 30 kD thiol-rich antigen (63). Although it is still primarily a research tool, direct PCR of stool specimens can differentiate *E. histolytica* from *E. dispar* rapidly. In addition to determining which patients should be treated, this technique has the potential to separate strains for epidemiological studies (64).

Serology

Serologic testing is still a key test for the diagnosis of invasive amebiasis. More than 90% of patients develop antibodies to *E. histolytica*, which can be detected by ELISA (65), indirect hemagglutination (66), counterimmuno-electrophoresis (67), or agar gel diffusion (68). Diagnosis of acute amebiasis based on a positive IHA titer may be problematic as antibody may be detectable as long as ten years after acute disease (69). In contrast, ELISA, AGD, and CIE tend to revert to negative within months, so a positive titer usually reflects acute disease. The titer of antibody correlates with the length of infection, not the severity of disease (28). Therefore, up to 10% of patients presenting acutely with an amebic liver abscess may be seronegative, but develop detectable antibody within a few days to two weeks (28). Even asymptomatic patients colonized with *E. histolytica* develop antibody responses (10). Therefore, serologic testing can be very useful in determining if an asymptomatic cyst passer is harboring *E. histolytica* if stool ELISA or PCR is not available. Detection of sIgA in saliva correlated well with serum ELISA and may be a good noninvasive screening method (70).

Radiographic Studies

Noninvasive radiographic studies are important in the early diagnosis of amebic liver abscess. Ultrasound examination typically shows a round or oval hypoechoic area with wall echoes (71). Computerized tomography (Fig. 3) and MRI are also very sensitive. The size, location, and number of abscesses also help determine appropriate treatment. More than 80% of patients with symptoms for more than ten days have a single abscess in the right lobe of the liver (28). Multiple lesions occur in up to 50% of patients who present acutely, and aspiration may be required to differentiate an amebic from a pyogenic abscess (45). Other potential indications for percutaneous drainage include left lobe abscesses, which may rupture into the pericardium, failure to respond to medical therapy in 72 hours, and imminent rupture with abscesses larger than 12 cm (72). Abscesses are slow to resolve and may actually increase in size despite successful therapy (71). Thus, there is no indication to reimage a patient acutely unless complications develop. The ultrasound returns to normal within six months in 2/3 of patients, but may take as long as one year in others (71).

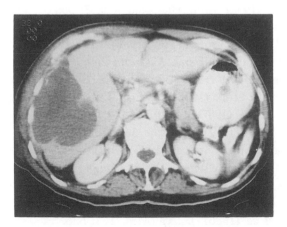

Figure 3. CT scan of patient with amebic liver abscess. A large, right lobe liver abscess which ruptured into the peritoneum is seen in a patient who presented with fever and severe right upper quadrant pain.

Barium enemas are relatively contraindicated in amebic colitis because of the risk of perforation, however, amebomas are usually detected only by the use of this technique to evaluate abdominal masses.

Conclusions

The diagnosis of invasive amebic disease must be considered in any febrile patient, particularly with gastrointestinal symptoms or travel to endemic areas. The clinical diagnosis can be confirmed by noninvasive radiologic studies, serology, and identification of E. *histolytica* from stools or liver abscesses. Advances in diagnostic techniques which include antigen detection and PCR now allow direct, rapid identification of E. *histolytica* from clinical specimens and offer the opportunity to initiate early therapy for this readily treatable parasitic infection.

References

1. Walsh JA (1988). *Amebiasis. Human Infection by Entamoeba histolytica*, ed. Ravdin JI (John Wiley and Sons , New York).
2. Ravdin JI (1995). *Clin. Infect. Dis.* **20**: 1453.
3. Reed SL (1992). *Clin. Infect. Dis.* **14**: 385.
4. Bruckner DA (1992). *Clin. Microbiol. Rev.* **5**: 356.
5. Nanda R, *et al.* (1984). *Lancet* **2**: 301.
6. Gathiram V and Jackson TFHG (1985). *Lancet* **1**: 719.
7. Reed SL, *et al.* (1991). *Am. J. Med.* **90**: 269.
8. Allason-Jones E, *et al.* (1988). *Br. Med. J.* **297**: 654.
9. Allason-Jones E, *et al.* (1986). *N. Eng. J. Med.* **315**: 353.
10. Gathiram V, *et al.* (1987). *S. Afr. Med. J.* **72**: 669.
11. Adams EB, *et al.* (1977). *Medicine* **56**: 315.
12. Chadee K and Meerovitch E (1985). *Am. J. Pathol.* **119**: 485.
13. Chadee K and Meerovitch E (1984). *Am. J. Pathol.* **117**: 71.
14. Takeuchi A, *et al.* (1975). *Am. J. Trop. Med. Hyg.* **24**: 34.
15. Seydel KB, *et al.* (1997). *Infect. Immun.* **65**: 1631.
16. Keene WE, *et al.* (1986). *J. Exp. Med.* **163**: 536.
17. Reed SL, *et al.* (1989). *J. Clin. Microbiol.* **27**: 2772.
18. Chadee K, *et al.* (1987). *J. Clin. Invest.* **80**: 1245.
19. McCoy JJ, *et al.* (1994). *Infect. Immun.* **62**: 3045.

20. Long-Krug SA, *et al.* (1985). *J. Infect. Dis.* **152**: 536.
21. Leippe M, *et al.* (1991). *Proc. Natl. Acad. Sci. USA* **88**: 7659.
22. Jansson A, *et al.* (1994). *Science* **263**: 1440.
23. Eckmann L, *et al.* (1995). *J. Clin. Invest.* **95**: 55.
24. Yu Y, *et al.* (1997). *Gastro* **112**: 1536.
25. Fuchs G, *et al.* (1988). *Amebiasis. Human infection by Entamoeba histolytica,* ed. Ravdin JI (John Wiley and Sons, New York).
26. Aristizabal H, *et al.* (1991). *World J. Surg.* **15**: 216.
27. Patel AS, *et al.* (1989). *J. Clin. Gastroenterol.* **11**: 407.
28. Katzenstein D, *et al.* (1982). *Medicine* **61**: 237.
29. Irusen EM, *et al.* (1992). *Clin. Infect. Dis.* **14**: 889.
30. Reed SL, *et al.* (1990). *J. Clin. Invest.* **86**: 1815.
31. Braga L, *et al.* (1992). *J. Clin. Invest.* **90**: 1131.
32. Harriman GR, *et al.* (1982). *J. Exp. Med.* **156**: 1235.
33. Joiner KA, *et al.* (1984). *Ann. Rev. Immunol.* **2**: 461.
34. Klatskin G (1946). *Ann. Int. Med.* **25**: 601.
35. Adams EB and MacLeod IN (1977). *Medicine* **56**: 325.
36. Rode H, *et al.* (1978). *S. Afr. J. Surg.* **16**: 131.
37. Cameron EWJ (1978). *Chest* **75**: 647.
38. Vickers PJ, *et al.* (1982). *Int. Surg.* **67**: 427.
39. Ibarra-Perez C (1981). *Chest* **79**: 672.
40. Ibarra-Perez C and Selman-Lama M (1977). *Amer. J. Surg.* **134**: 283.
41. Verghese M, *et al.* (1979). *J. Thorac. Cardiovasc. Surg.* **78**: 757.
42. Eggleston FC, *et al.* (1978). *Surgery* **83**: 536.
43. Ibarra-Perez C, *et al.* (1972). *J. Thorac. Cardiovasc. Surg.* **64**: 11.
44. Adeyemo AO, *et al.* (1984). *J. Roy. Soc. Med.* **77**: 17.
45. Thompson JE, *et al.* (1985). *Rev. Infect. Dis.* **7**: 171.
46. Orbison JA, *et al.* (1951). *Medicine* **30**: 247.
47. Kean BH, *et al.* (1956). *Ann. Int. Med.* **44**: 831.
48. Schmutzhard F, *et al.* (1986). *Eur. Neurol.* **25**: 161.
49. Ohnishi K, *et al.* (1994). *Am. J. Trop. Med. Hyg.* **51**: 180.
50. Kirsh D and Diaz-Rivera S (1943). *Am. J. Med. Sci.* **206**: 372.
51. Andrew WK and Thomas RG (1981). *S. A. Med. J.* **59**: 571.
52. Heinz KPW (1973). *S. A. Med. J.* **47**: 1795.
53. Purpon I, *et al.* (1967). *J. Urol.* **98**: 372.
54. Veliath AJ, *et al.* (1987). *Int. J. Gynaecol. Obstet.* **25**: 24.
55. DeBakey ME and Jordan GL (1977). *Surg. Clin. N. Amer.* **57**: 325.
56. WHO/Pan America Health Organization Expert Consultation on Amebiasis, *WHO Weekly Epidem. Rec.* **72**: 97.

57. Sargeaunt PG, *et al.* (1978). *Trans. R. Soc. Trop. Med. Hyg.* **72**: 164.
58. Abd-Alla MD, *et al.* (1993). *J. Clin. Microbiol.* **1**: 2845.
59. Haque R, *et al.* (1995). *J. Clin. Microbiol.* **33**: 2558.
60. Katzwinkel-Wladarsch S, *et al.* (1994). *Am. J. Trop. Med. Hyg.* **51**: 115.
61. Soto Acuna R, *et al.* (1993). *Am. J. Trop. Med. Hyg.* **48**: 58.
62. Clark CB, *et al.* (1991). *Mol. Biochem. Parasitol.* **49**: 297.
63. Tachibana H, *et al.* (1991). *J. Clin. Microbiol.* **29**: 2234.
64. Clark CG, *et al.* (1993). *Exp. Parasit.* **77**: 450.
65. Sathar MA, *et al.* (1990). *J. Clin. Microbiol.* **28**: 332.
66. Krupp IM (1970). *Am. J. Trop. Med. Hyg.* **19 (1)**: 57.
67. Krupp IM (1974). *Am. J. Trop. Med. Hyg.* **23**: 27.
68. Powell SJ, *et al* (1965). *Lancet* **2**: 602.
69. Healy GR (1986). *Infect. Dis.* **8**: 239.
70. del Muro R, *et al.* (1990). *J. Infect. Dis.* **162**: 1360.
71. Ralls PW, *et al.* (1983). *Radiology* **149**: 541.
72. Ralph P, *et al.* (1975). *J. Immunol.* **114**: 898.
73. DeBakey ME and Ochsner A (1951). *Int. Abstr. Surg.* **92**: 209.

Chapter 6

Treatment

DR Pillai, JS Keystone and KC Kain

Tropical Disease Unit, EN G-224
Toronto General Hospital, 200 Elizabeth Street
Toronto, ON, Canada, M5G 2C4
E-mail: kkain@torhosp.toronto.on.ca

The treatment of amebiasis has two fundamental objectives: (i) to cure invasive disease at both intestinal and extra-intestinal sites and (ii) to eliminate the passage of cysts from the bowel lumen. Metronidazole has emerged as the drug of choice for the treatment of invasive disease. Other 5-nitroimidazole derivatives such as tinidazole, ornidazole, and secnidazole, available outside of North America, may be equally efficacious. Several lumenal agents are available to eradicate cyst passage. Diloxanide furoate is the preferred agent but is not readily available. Other effective agents include paromomycin and iodoquinol. One complicating factor in the use of these agents has been the overwhelming evidence that there exists a morphologically identical but genetically distinct non-pathogenic species, *Entomoeba dispar*. This organism does not cause disease and therefore requires no chemotherapy. Controlled trials with antigen detection kits and PCR-based assays that can distinguish E. *histolytica* from E. *dispar* are in progress. However, until these techniques are fully evaluated and widely available, treatment of asymptomatic cyst passers in non-endemic is suggested. Treatment of asymptomatic cyst passers in areas where E. *histolytica* is endemic remains a futile public health policy due to high rates of re-infection. In addition to chemotherapy, drainage of amebic liver abscesses using fine needle aspiration, guided by ultrasound or computed tomography, is a useful therapeutic intervention when (i) abscesses are extremely large and there is danger of imminent rupture, (ii) medical therapy has failed, (iii) a left lobe abscess threatens to rupture into the pericardium, or (iv) immediate symptomatic relief is required. Surgical intervention is reserved for toxic megacolon complicating amebic colitis or in cases where hepatic abscesses have ruptured into the peritoneal cavity.

Treatment

Non-Invasive Disease (Asymptomatic Cyst/Trophozoite Passers)

Most asymptomatic individuals diagnosed with "amebiasis", based on stool microscopy, will in fact be infected with the harmless commensal *E. dispar*. Preliminary data indicate that ELISA and PCR tests can distinguish *E. dispar* from *E. histolytica* (1–5). Amebic serology may be an alternative strategy for the diagnosis *of E. histolytica* in non-endemic areas, since several studies have shown that antibodies develop only during infection with *E. histolytica*, even in those who are asymptomatic (6–8). In these studies, negative serology virtually ruled out *E. histolytica* infection. However, a recent study of German travelers showed a disturbingly low sensitivity for amebic serology among those infected with *E. histolytica* (8). One possible factor for the poor results may be the fact that antibodies are often not detectable during the first week of infection. Furthermore, serology is of limited use in endemic areas since antibodies may persist for years after infection. Therefore, unless serology is readily available, or until new antigen or PCR-based assays are fully evaluated and available, all asymptomatic cyst passers and excreters of trophozoites should be treated with a lumen-active agent alone (see Table 1).

Diloxanide furoate (Furamide) is the preferred agent for eradicating intralumenal cyst passage (9). A 10-day course has an 85% success rate in

Table 1. Treatment of the asymptomatic cyst passer.

Drug	Adult dosage (po)	Pediatric dosage (po)
Diloxanide furoate[ψ] (Furamide)	500 mg tid × 10 days	10 mg/kg/day × 10 days (max 1500 mg/day)
Paromomycin (Humatin)	30 mg/kg/day × 7 days	25 mg/kg/day[Φ] × 7 days (max 2 g/day)
Iodoquinol (Yodoxin)	650 mg tid × 20 days	30–40 mg/kg/days[Φ] × 20 days (max 2 g/day)

[ψ]In U.S.A. available only through the Centers for Disease Control: telephone (404) 639-3670 or (404) 639-3356 days and (404) 639-2888 nights and emergencies. In Canada: Bureau of Pharmaceutical Assessment, Health Protection Branch, Ottawa (613) 941-2108.

[Φ]Administered in three divided doses.

eliminating the organism. Less than 10% of the oral dose is excreted in the feces, but sufficient amounts of the active form accumulate in the colonic lumen. The remainder is hydrolyzed within the intestinal mucosa, absorbed, and ultimately excreted in the urine. Treatment is regarded as successful if the stools remain free of cysts and trophozoites for one month. Due to the irregular excretion pattern of the organism in stool, several specimens should be evaluated to document cure. Diloxanide is relatively nontoxic; occasional mild gastrointestinal symptoms and increased flatulence are the most frequent side effects (10). Treatment is best deferred, however, until after the first trimester of pregnancy. This drug is available only through the Centers for Disease Control and Prevention (CDC) in the USA and Bureau of Pharmaceutical Assessment, Health Protection Branch (HPB) in Canada.

An alternative and equally efficacious lumenal agent is paromomycin (Humatin), an aminoglycoside which is not absorbed from the gasrointestinal tract and is safe in pregnancy (11–15). Diarrhea and abdominal cramps are the only significant side effects (16). Iodoquinol (Yodoxin) is also marketed in North America and is equally effective as diloxanide furoate but requires a longer treatment course (20 days compared to 10 days for diloxanide and 7 days for paromomycin). In addition to gastrointestinal side effects, iodoquinol may interfere with thyroid function due to its high iodine content. Rare dose-related neurotoxicity, such as optic neuritis, has been reported with prolonged drug use or inappropriately high dosage (17). As with diloxanide, follow up stool examinations are essential to monitor the success of treatment since failure rates occur in 10–15% of individuals treated with any of the lumenal agents. In vitro studies with bacitracin zinc suggest that it may also be useful as an alternative non-toxic lumenal agent (18). Notably, metronidazole (Flagyl) or its counterpart 5-nitroimidazole derivatives should not be used to treat the asymptomatic cyst or trophozoite passer since these drugs are active in tissue infection but often fail to eradicate organisms from the lumen.

Invasive Disease

Intestinal sites (amebic colitis)

Metronidazole (Flagyl) is the drug of choice for patients with acute and chronic forms of invasive intestinal disease including ameboma. Table 2 summarizes alternative treatment strategies. Metronidazole is a

Table 2. Treatment of invasive disease — amebic colitis.*

Drug	Adult dosage (po)	Pediatric dosage (po)
Metronidazole[ѱ] (Flagyl)	750 mg tid × 5–10 days or 2.5 g once daily × 3 days	30–50 mg/kg day[Φ] × 10 days (max 2250 mg/day)
Tinidazole[δ] (Fasigyn)	2 g once daily × 3 days	50 mg/kg/day[Φ] × 3 days
Alternative: Dehydroemetine[ς] (Mebadin)	1–1.5 mg/kg/day IM × 5 days (max 90 mg/day)	1–1.5 mg/kg/day[Φ] × 20 days (max 90 mg/day)

*Treatment of invasive disease is followed by a complete course of a lumenal agent as described in Table 1 for the asymptomatic cyst passer.

[ς]In U.S.A.: available only through the Centers for Disease Control: telephone (404) 639-3670 or (404) 639-3356 days and (404) 639-2888 nights and emergencies. In Canada: Bureau of Pharmaceutical Assessment, Health Protection Branch, Ottawa (613) 941-2108.

[Φ]Administered in three divided doses.

[δ]Marketed outside of U.S.A. and Canada.

[ѱ]May be administered intravenously if patient unable to take by mouth (500 mg IV every 6 h × 5–10 days).

5-nitroimidazole derivative with anti-microbial activity against some anaerobic bacteria as well as protozoa such as *E. histolytica* and *Giardia intestinalis*. Metronidazole is almost completely absorbed following oral administration. It is highly efficacious with 90% cure rates in many well-controlled studies (20–21). Despite widespread use, *E. histolytica* resistance to metronidazole has not yet become a clinical problem. It is important to note however, that the complement of genes associated with multi-drug resistance and the drug-efflux mechanism do exist in this organism (22). Although most authorities recommend that amebic colitis be treated for 7 to 10 days, studies indicate that 2.4 g of metronidazole given p.o. once daily for 3 days is equally effective (23). The use of metronidazole during pregnancy has been controversial with one study suggesting teratogenic effects when used in the first trimester and others suggesting safety in pregnancy (24–25). A comparison of one cohort of 1,000 patients who received the drug with those who did not showed no adverse effects to the fetus (26). Indeed, therapy during pregnancy is warranted for invasive amebic disease because of the increased risk of fulminant amebiasis and severe complications.

Common side effects of metronidazole are primarily gastrointestinal (nausea, headache, metallic taste, abdominal discomfort) and central nervous system (headache, dizziness, and drowsiness) in origin (27). Other side effects include dark coloured urine, urticaria, and transient neutropenia (28). Patients should avoid alcoholic beverages due to metronidazole's disulfiram-like properties (29). The drug is also available for intravenous administration in patients unable to take oral medications. Since metronidazole usually fails to eliminate intestinal carriage, a lumen-active agent should always be given in conjuction for any form of invasive disease (amebic colitis or amebic liver abscess — see next section) whether or not parasites are detected on stool examination (23). To reduce the likelihood of additive side effects, these drugs may be given sequentially (see Tables 2 and 3).

Outside of the United States and Canada, tinidazole (Fasigyn), a 5-nitroimidazole derivative, is the preferred drug for treatment of invasive disease (20–21). It is generally associated with fewer gastrointestinal side effects. As with metronidazole, a lumen-active agent must also be administered.

Tetracycline or erythromycin followed by a lumenal agent are effective alternatives for patients with mild amebic colitis who are unable to tolerate metronidazole. However, these regimens do not eradicate parasites in the liver and care must be taken to assess the patient for hepatic involvement.

Table 3. Treatment of amebic liver abscess[*].

Drug	Adult dosage (po)	Pediatric dosage (po)
Metronidazole[ᵚ] (Flagyl)	750 mg tid × 5–10 days or 2.5 g orally once	30–50 mg/kg/day[Φ] × 5–10 days
Alternative: Dehydroemetine[ᶴ] (Mebadin)	1–1.5 mg/kg/day IM × 5 days (maximum 90 mg/day)	1–1.5 mg/kg/day[Φ] × 20 days (maximum 90 mg/day)

[*]Treatment of invasive disease is followed by a complete course of a lumenal agent as described in Table 1 for the asymptomatic cyst passer.
[ᶴ]In U.S.A. available only through the Centers for Disease Control: telephone (404) 639-3670 or (404) 639-3356 days and (404) 639-2888 nights and emergencies. In Canada: Bureau of Pharmaceutical Assessment, Health Protection Branch, Ottawa (613) 941-2108.
[Φ]Administered in three divided doses.
[ᵚ]May be administered intravenously if patient unable to take by mouth (500 mg IV every 6 h × 5–10 days).

An alternative drug is dehydroemetine (Mebadin) which is rapidly amebicidal in tissues but not the lumen (30). This drug is associated with significant gastrointestinal, cardiac, and neuromuscular side effects. Neuromuscular reactions include muscle weakness and pain, stiffness of the limbs and neck. Cardiotoxicity results in ECG changes (T-wave flattening or inversion), fall in blood pressure, and tachycardia (30–31). There is no clear evidence that combining dehydroemetine with metronidazole is more efficacious than metronidazole alone in the treatment of invasive amebiasis. Dehydroemetine is only available in North America with the authorization of the CDC or HPB. As in asymptomatic cyst passers, follow-up stool examinations should be performed 2–4 weeks after the completion of therapy to detect treatment failures.

Intestinal perforation during amebic colitis is best managed with therapy consisting of antiamebic and antibacterial agents. Surgical resection (usually in the form of total colectomy) is generally reserved for patients with toxic megacolon.

Extra-Intestinal Sites

Outside of the gastrointestinal tract, *E. histolytica* may metastasize to the liver, lung, brain, and skin. The most common site of tissue invasion is the liver. Patients with amebic liver abscess (ALA) generally present with fever, weight loss, abdominal pain, and hepatic tenderness. The diagnosis is established by demonstrating a space-occupying lesion in the liver through either ultrasonography, CT or MRI scan (32–35). Amebic serology is positive in 99% of patients, but may occasionally be negative within the first week of symptom onset (35).

ALA and invasion of other sites can usually be managed by medical therapy alone (see Fig. 1 & Table 3). The preferred drug is metronidazole followed by an agent to eradicate intralumenal infection. In uncomplicated mild to moderate disease, single dose therapy with 2.5 g of metronidazole has been effective, and provides an alternative to those patients who cannot tolerate the standard 5 to 10 day regimen (23). Chloroquine is known to be a potent amebicide in hepatic tissue alone and some clinicians have recommended the addition of chloroquine to metronidazole when treating critically ill patients. However, there are no well-controlled trials to support the use of combination therapy.

Percutaneous drainage of liver abscess should be reserved for patients who are not responding to medical therapy or who have large abscesses

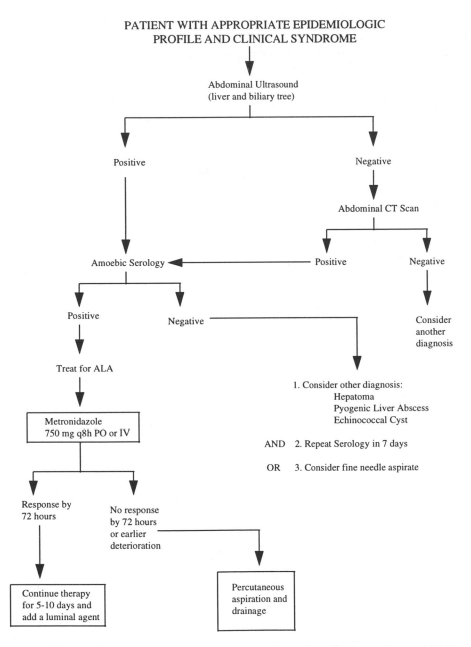

Figure 1. Algorithm for the evaluation and treatment of amebic liver abscess (ALA). CT, computed tomography.

Table 4. Indications for aspiration of amebic liver abscess.

1. Failure of medical therapy (no response within 3 days to metronidazole).
2. Left lobe abscesses with danger of rupture into the pericardium.
3. Large abscesses where rupture is believed to be imminent.
4. To rule out pyogenic abscess when there are multiple lesions.
5. For prompt symptomatic relief of severe pain.

which threaten to rupture (36–37). In addition, left lobe abscesses can potentially rupture into the pericardium and therefore require surgical drainage if percutaneous access to the abscess is not possible. Aspiration may provide prompt symptomatic relief to those with severe right upper quadrant abdominal pain.

There is some recent evidence that ultrasound- and computer tomography-guided drainage in combination with intralesional chemotherapy improves outcomes in ALA, compared to medical therapy alone, or medical therapy with surgical drainage (38). However, in general, drainage is recommended only for the complicated case of ALA (see Table 4). The abscess cavity often resolves slowly over several months as determined by ultrasonography and up to 20% of patients will have a permanent hepatic cystic cavity after the completion of therapy (39–40). Amebic antibodies as determined by indirect hemagglutination and ELISA may take from 2 to 10 years to disappear after successful treatment.

References

1. Haque RK., Kress K, Wood S, Jackson T, Lyerly D, Wilkins T and Petri WA (1993). *J. Infect. Dis.* **167**: 247–249.
2. Acuna-Soto R, Samuelson J, de Girolami P, Zarate L, Millan-Velasco F, Schoolnick G and Wirth D (1993). *Am. J. Trop. Med. Hyg.* **48**: 58–70.
3. Britten D, Wilson SM, McNerney R, Moody AH, Chiodini PL and Ackers JP (1997). *J. Clin. Micro.* **35 (5)**: 1108–1111.
4. Troll H, Marti H and Weiss N (1997). *J. Clin. Micro.* **35 (7)**: 1701–1705.
5. Pillai DR, Britten D, Ackers JP, Ravdin JI and Kain KC (1997). *Mol. Biochem. Parasitol.* **87**: 101–105.
6. Jackson TFHG, Gathiram V and Simjee AE (1985). *Lancet* **1**: 716–719.
7. Ravdin JI, Jackson TF, Petri WA Jr, *et al.* (1990). *J. Infect. Dis.* **162**: 768–772.

8. Walderich B, Weber A and Knobloch J (1997). *Am. J. Trop. Med. Hyg.* **57 (1)**: 70–74.

9. McAuley JB, Herwaldt BL, Stokes SL, Becher JA, Roberts JM, Michelson MK and Juranek DD (1992). *Clin. Infect. Dis.* **15**: 464–468.

10. Wolfe MS (1973). *JAMA.* **224**: 1601–1604.

11. Botero DR (1964). *Trans. R. Soc. Trop. Med. Hyg.* **58**: 419–421.

12. Suchak NG, Satoskar RS and Sheth UK (1962). *Am. J. Trop. Med. & Hyg.* **11**: 330–332.

13. Woodruff AW and Bell S (1967). *Trans. R. Soc. Trop. Med. Hyg.* **61**: 435–439.

14. Carter CH, Bayles A and Thompson PE (1968). *Am. J. Trop. Med. & Hyg.* **11**: 448–451.

15. McAuley JB and Juranek DD (1992). *Clin. Infect. Dis.* **15**: 551–552.

16. Keusch GT, Troncale FJ and Buchanan RD (1970). *Arch. Intern. Med.* **125**: 273–276.

17. Fisher AK, Walter FG and Szabo S (1993). *J. of Toxicology — Clinical Toxicology.* **31 (1)**: 113–120.

18. Andrews BJ and Bjorvatn B (1994). *Trans. R. Soc. Trop. Med. Hyg.* **88**: 98–100.

19. Bassilly S, Farid Z, El-Masry NA and Mikhail EM (1987). *J. Trop. Med. Hyg.* **90**: 9–12.

20. Simjee AE, Gathiram V, Jackson TFGH and Khan BFY (1985). *S. Afr. Med. J.* **68**: 923–924.

21. Samuelson JC, Burke A and Courval JM (1992). *Antimicrob. Agents & Chemotherapy* **36 (11)**: 2392–2397.

22. Irusen EM, Jackson TFHG and Simjee AE (1992). *Clin. Infect. Dis.* **14**: 889–893.

23. Briggs GG, Freeman RK, Yaffe SJ (eds) (1994). Drugs in pregnancy and lactation. A reference guide to fetal and neonatal risk (4th Ed.). Baltimore: Williams & Wilkins, pp. 585–587.

24. Burtin P, Taddio A, Aribumu O, Einanan TR and Koren G (1995). *Amer. J. Obst. & Gyn.* **172 (2 Pt 1)**: 525–529.

25. Piper JM, Mitchel EF and Ray WA (1993). *Obst. & Gyn.* **82 (3)**: 348–352.

26. Lau AH, Lam NP and Piscitelli SS. *Clin. Pharmacokinet.* **23**: 328–364.

27. Roe FJC (1985). *Scand. J. Inf. Dis.* **46**: 72–81.

28. Rothstein E and Clancy DD (1969). *N. Eng. J. Med.* **280**: 1006–1007.

29. Powell SW, Wilmost AJ, McLeod IN, *et al.* (1965). *Ann. Trop. Med. Parasitol.* **59**: 208–209.

30. Salem HH and Abd-Rabbo H (1964). *J. Trop. Med. Hyg.* **67**: 137–141.
31. Sukov, *et al.* (1980). *Amer. J. Roentgenology* **134 (5)**: 911–915.
32. Wagner-Manslau C, Reiser M and Lukas P (1985). *Radiologe.* **25 (12)**: 597–598.
33. Elizondo G, Weissleder R, Stark DD, Todd LE, Compton C, Wittenberg J and Ferrucci JT (1987). *Radiology.* **165**: 795–800.
34. Nordestgaard AG, Stapleford L, Worthen N, Bongard FS and Klein SR (1992). *The Amer. Surgeon* **58 (5)**: 315–320.
35. Sharma MP, Rai RR, Acharya SK, Ray JCS and Tandon BN (1989). *Br. Med. J.* **299**: 1308–1309.
36. Ramani A, Ramani R, Kumar MS, Lakhkar BN and Kundaje GN (1993). *Postgrad. Med. J.* **69**: 381–383.
37. Filice C, Di Perri G, Strosselli M, Brunetti E, Dughetti S, van Thiel DH and Scotti-Foflieni C (1992). *Digest. Dis. & Sci.* **37 (2)**: 240–247.
38. Ralls PW, Quinn MF, Boswell Jr WD, *et al.* (1983). *Radiology.* **149**: 541–543.
39. Ahmed L, Salama ZA, El Rooby A and Strickland GT (1989). *Amer. J. Trop. Med Hyg.* **4**: 406–410.

Chapter 7

Prevention and Potential of New Interventions

SL Stanley, Jr

Department of Medicine and Molecular Microbiology
Washington, University School of Medicine
660 S. Euclid Avenue, St. Louis
MO, 63110 USA
E-mail: sstanley@im.wustl.edu

The persistence of amebiasis as a global health problem, despite the availability of effective treatment, has led to the search for vaccines to prevent amebiasis. Recent progress in this area has been facilitated by the application of recombinant technology. Recombinant vaccines containing epitopes derived from the serine rich *E. histolytica* protein (SREHP), the 170 kDa subunit of the galactose-inhibitable lectin, and a 29 kDa cysteine rich protein, have been tested and found to be protective in animal models of amebic liver abscess. Oral vaccines, utilizing amebic antigens either co-administered with some form of cholera toxin, or expressed in attenuated strains of *Salmonella* or *Vibrio cholera*, have also been developed and tested in animals for mucosal immunogenicity. These new vaccine preparations show promise, but there are unanswered questions regarding the duration of immunity, and, as yet, the safety, immunogenicity, and efficacy of these vaccines in humans has not been established.

Introduction

Amebiasis remains a significant threat to public health in a number of countries around the world. In Mexico, for example, more than 8% of the population are seropositive for amebiasis, consistent with a previous episode of invasive disease (1). Over the past century, improvements in sanitation have greatly reduced amebiasis in much of Europe, the United States, Australasia, and Canada, but it is unlikely that these public health interventions will be available to all the world's population in the near future. Therefore, other approaches to prevent amebiasis need to be considered. Vaccines can be a cost-effective and potent approach to disease prevention, and even disease eradication. Effective vaccines are now available against a variety of bacterial and viral pathogens, but no vaccine against a protozoan or helminth parasite has yet gained acceptance for widespread use in humans. This reflects the fact that parasitic diseases can pose special challenges for vaccine development, including the presence of complex life cycles, with multiple, antigenically diverse stages and intermediate hosts, animal reservoirs of disease, and sophisticated methods of immune evasion. In addition, many protozoan parasites reside within host cells, reducing their susceptibility to host immune defenses. However, *E. histolytica* appears to present few of these challenges to vaccine development. The life cycle is simple, there are no intermediate hosts, and it is an extracellular parasite. *E. histolytica* may possess strategies for immune evasion (see chapter 4), but one of the most difficult to overcome for vaccine development, antigenic variation, has not been detected in *E. histolytica*. For these reasons, a vaccine to prevent amebiasis may be more readily achievable than vaccines against other protozoan parasites. Since man is the definitive host, the development of a vaccine that effectively prevented *E. histolytica* infection in susceptible humans could potentially eradicate this parasite.

Three paradigms have guided recent work on vaccine development for amebiasis. The first is that protective immunity to amebiasis can be achieved. There is convincing data from animal studies in support of this concept. As detailed below, experiments in several different animal models of amebic liver abscess have indicated that prior infection, vaccination, and passive immunisation, can provide protection against a challenge infection. Unfortunately, there are few human studies addressing this concept. A single epidemiologic study indicated that individuals who had a prior episode of amebic liver abscess had a lower rate of subsequent amebic liver abscess than a historical control group consisting of previously uninfected individuals (2). While far from definitive, the combination of the data from animal studies, and the limited experience in humans, provides evidence for the existence of protective immunity to amebiasis.

The second paradigm is that recombinant amebic antigens offer advantages over either native *E. histolytica* antigens, or inactivated/attenuated parasites for amebic vaccines. Because *E. histolytica* trophozoites are relatively expensive to grow in large quantities, and purification of native proteins can be time consuming and costly, basing vaccines on recombinant amebic antigens obtained by prokaryotic expression systems may save time and money. With recombinant technology, one can produce truncated proteins/peptides that contain protective epitopes and exclude other "extraneous" regions of the target antigen. As discussed below, this property has been especially important in the case of one of the major amebic vaccine candidates, where immunisation with the whole native molecule can result in protective immune responses in some vaccinated animals, but exacerbate disease in other recipients (3). Recombinant amebic antigens can be expressed in vaccine delivery vectors, such as attenuated vaccine strains of salmonellae and *Vibrio cholerae*, offering the possibility of combination vaccines designed to prevent multiple enteric infections. This feature has figured prominently in many of the new designs for amebiasis vaccines. Finally, recombinant amebic antigens can be genetically fused to other biologically active molecules to improve their immunogenicity. The fusion of amebic antigens to components of cholera toxin has been another prominent strategy in amebic vaccine development. Because of these advantages, most of the recent studies on amebic vaccines have utilised recombinant antigens, and there is little recent work on native antigens or attenuated/killed *E. histolytica*-based vaccines. However, there have been no "head to head" comparisons of recombinant-antigen based vaccines and whole *E. histolytica* vaccines, and the important question of whether there are any differences in efficacy between these approaches remains unanswered.

The third paradigm is that amebic vaccines should stimulate mucosal immune responses to *E. histolytica*. Amebiasis begins with *E. histolytica* trophozoites attaching to human intestinal epithelial cells. Amebic invasion into intestinal mucosa, the penetration into submucosal tissue, and the establishment of extraintestinal disease (most commonly amebic liver abscess) all depend upon this first attachment step. The induction of mucosal antibodies, capable of blocking amebic adherence to intestinal epithelial cells, could abort the establishment of infection, and thereby prevent intestinal and extraintestinal disease. Clinical support for this hypothesis has come from experiments showing that IgA antibodies isolated from the saliva of patients with amebic intestinal disease can block amebic adherence to target cells (4). In addition, it has been demonstrated that rats vaccinated with the native 220 kDa galactose-inhibitable lectin and the B subunit of cholera toxin administered by direct inoculation into the rat's Peyer's patches, develop mucosal IgA anti-lectin antibodies capable of inhibiting amebic adherence to mammalian cells (5). Whether mucosal anti-amebic antibodies induced by vaccination can actually prevent the establishment of infection in vivo has been harder to establish. This reflects the fact that there have been few, if any, reliable animal models of intestinal amebiasis. This may change in the near future, as a model of intestinal amebiasis in the C3H/ HeJ mouse has recently been reported (6), and others have established intestinal infection by the novel approach of inoculating *E. histolytica* trophozoites into human intestinal xenografts transplanted into severe combined immunodeficient (SCID) mice (7). However, these methods are still new, and to date almost all recent vaccine studies have looked at protection from amebic liver abscess, since gerbils, hamsters, and severe combined immunodeficient (SCID) mice provide reproducible animal models of this disease. Despite the lack of extensive experimental validation for the concept that the induction of mucosal immune responses is desirable for amebic vaccines, much of the recent work in amebiasis vaccines has focused on antigen delivery systems designed to stimulate mucosal antibody responses to amebic antigens. Consistent with this concept, the two *E. histolytica* antigens selected for most of the vaccine studies, the serine rich *E. histolytica* protein (SREHP) and the 170 kDa subunit of the galactose-inhibitable lectin, are surface antigens, and in vitro studies have shown that antibodies to these antigens can block amebic adherence to target cells (8–10).

The importance of these three paradigms in amebic vaccine development will be apparent in the subsequent sections, which will summarise the limited work on native antigen and whole trophozoite-based amebic vaccines, provide a detailed analysis of the vaccine work on recombinant versions of the SREHP molecule and the galactose-inhibitable lectin, briefly discuss other vaccine candidates, and conclude with a discussion of the possible directions for future vaccine studies.

Complex Native Amebic Antigen and Whole Trophozoite-based Vaccines

Early experimental studies on protective immunity to amebiasis focused on whether immunity to disease arises after experimental infection. In one of the first studies in this field, dogs were experimentally infected per anum with *E. histolytica*, than following chemotherapy, or natural clearance of infection, were re-challenged with amebic trophozoites. Only 17% of the previously infected dogs developed intestinal disease after the second challenge, consistent with the development of a protective immune response (11). A similar study looked at drug terminated amebic liver abscess in hamsters, and found significant levels of protection from subsequent hepatic challenge in hamsters that had a previous episode of amebic liver abscess (12). Other investigators looked at the resistance to *E. histolytica* cecal infection in guinea pigs that were first inoculated with a "noninvasive" strain of *E. histolytica*. Prior infection with this strain provided some protection against subsequent intracecal challenge with a virulent strain of *E. histolytica* (13). This study provides some rationale for considering whether experimentally induced infection with *E. dispar*, which shares a number of antigens with *E. histolytica*, might provide protective immunity against *E. histolytica* infection, or whether chemically or genetically-attenuated live *E. histolytica* trophozoites might also serve as an effective oral vaccine. The newfound ability to axenically culture *E. dispar*, and the growing number of molecular tools for altering or suppressing gene expression in *E. histolytica* make both of these approaches testable (14). One technical obstacle for an attenuated *E. histolytica* trophozoite vaccine would be how infection would be established in the vaccine recipient, since trophozoites are quite fragile, and do not survive the acidity of the stomach, making oral delivery difficult. Feeding of cysts could be effective, but to date it has been impossible to get *E. histolytica* trophozoites to encyst in culture, providing a barrier to using a laboratory-derived strain. One recent approach to studying the immune response to whole amebic trophozoites has been to orally challenge animals with glutaraldehyde-fixed *E. histolytica* trophozoites (15). Both mice and rats reportedly develop systemic and mucosal antiamebic immune responses after intragastric inoculation of glutaraldehyde-fixed ameba. Interestingly, in addition to IgA antibodies, IgE was detected in cecal contents, and eosinophils were present in the lamina propria of inoculated rats, suggesting oral challenge with glutaraldehyde-fixed trophozoites induces a hypersensitivity reaction to amebic antigens. Whether this would be a protective response, or potentially damaging to the host upon rechallenge with live ameba, was not addressed in these studies.

A number of investigators have been able to induce protective immunity to amebic liver abscess and intestinal disease in small animal models of amebiasis by parenteral immunisation with amebic antigens. Slightly more than one-third of 90 rats immunised subcutaneously with a soluble amebic antigen failed to develop cecal lesions after intestinal challenge with *E. histolytica* trophozoites, compared with only 8% of the control group (16). Intradermal inoculation of hamsters with live amebic trophozoites provided 90% protection from intrahepatic challenge with *E. histolytica* in one study, and the same investigators found intradermal vaccination with a crude amebic lysate or a high molecular weight fraction from that lysate also produced significant protection (17, 18). In another study, hamsters vaccinated intradermally with a mixture of amebic proteins and complete Freund's adjuvant developed smaller amebic liver abscesses following direct intrahepatic challenge with amebic trophozoites than control animals (19). Rabbits vaccinated with a soluble amebic antigen preparation and a mycobacterial glycolipid adjuvant showed complete protection against intrahepatic challenge and intracecal challenge with *E. histolytica* trophozoites (20). Taken as a whole, these studies provide some of the strongest evidence supporting the development of protective immunity to amebiasis. The obvious limitation to these studies is that in all cases the animals used are not naturally susceptible to infection with *E. histolytica*, hence the methods used to induce infections are artificial (e.g. direct intrahepatic or intracecal inoculation of amebic trophozoites). Thus, whether immunisation induces a protective immune response that would prevent infection of the gut and the liver through the natural route in a naturally susceptible host (e.g. humans) remains untested.

The Serine Rich *Entamoeba histolytica* Protein (SREHP)

The serine rich *E. histolytica* protein (SREHP) has been one of the most intensely studied candidate molecules for an amebiasis vaccine. The cDNA clone encoding the SREHP molecule was first isolated by differential screening of a *E. histolytica* cDNA library with mRNA from *Entamoeba moshkovskii* (strain Laredo), or mRNA from *E. histolytica* HM1 : IMSS strain, in a strategy was designed to isolate genes that were specifically expressed in *E. histolytica* and could play a role in virulence (9). One of the cDNA clones encoded a protein with a high number of serine residues (52 of 233 amino acids), hence the designation of serine rich *E. histolytica* protein (9). The other striking feature of the structure was the presence of multiple, tandemly repeated, highly conserved sequences of octapeptides and dodecapeptides. In this regard, the structural motif of the SREHP molecule resembles the circumsporozoite proteins of malaria, with a hydrophobic N-terminal region (signal sequence), followed by a region of highly charged amino acids consisting primarily of lysine, glutamic acid, and aspartic acid, leading to a series of tandemly repeated hydrophilic dodecapeptide or octapeptide sequences composed of serine, aspartic acid, threonine, proline, lysine, glutamic acid, asparagine, and alanine (9). This region is followed by a C-terminal hydrophobic domain consistent with a membrane insertion region. The full length SREHP cDNA clone encodes a peptide of approximately 25 kDa, but the native SREHP molecule was found to migrate at 47/52 kDa on SDS-PAGE due to the high proline content and hydrophilicity of the repeating units, and due to post-translational modifications of the SREHP molecule (21). *E. dispar* has a highly homologous gene to the *E. histolytica* SREHP, with nucleotide differences between the *E. histolytica* and *E. dispar* SREHP cDNA sequences primarily confined to the tandem repeats (22). Recently, the existence of a gene family (designated ARIEL) which encodes for SREHP-like molecules with high levels of sequence identity to SREHP in the regions flanking the tandem repeats, but some differences in the amino acid composition of the repeats (higher asparagine content), has been discovered (23).

SREHP is a surface membrane protein, but it has post-translational modifications which are more commonly seen in nuclear or cytoplasmic proteins (21). A number of the serine residues are phosphorylated, and SREHP possesses O-linked N-acetylglucosamine residues. SREHP appears to be anchored in the membrane by a C-terminal covalently-linked lipid, but does not appear to have a GPI anchor (21). The function of SREHP remains unknown. Antibodies to SREHP block amebic adherence to mammalian cells in vitro, but the isolated SREHP molecule shows no obvious adhesin properties (9, 10). SREHP can serve as a chemoattractant for *E. histolytica* trophozoites, but the physiologic relevance of this property is unknown (21).

SREHP is highly immunogenic (among individuals with amebic liver abscess more than 80% have serum antibodies to the SREHP molecule) and appears to possess a number of conserved epitopes (24). By synthesising a series of overlapping octapeptides that spanned the entire sequence of the SREHP molecule, and reacting them with serum samples from patients with amebic liver abscess, it was determined that most of the antibodies to SREHP bind epitopes within the dodecapeptide and octapeptide repeats of the molecules (25). Interestingly, there was no single epitope recognised by all the serum samples (25). SREHP appears to be the product of a single copy gene (26), and while the SREHP genes from different isolates of *E. histolytica* can differ in the number of dodecapeptide and octapeptide repeats encoded (this property is the basis of PCR tests that can differentiate between strains of *E. histolytica* (27)), no strain completely lacking sequences encoding the dodecapeptide repeat of SREHP has been described.

SREHP appears to possess a number of desirable properties for a candidate antigen for vaccine development. It is located on the surface of ameba, antibodies to SREHP can block amebic adherence to mammalian cells, and there are conserved SREHP epitopes in geographically and clinically diverse isolates of *E. histolytica*. The ability of antibodies to SREHP to provide protection against amebic liver abscess was first established in passive immunisation studies (10). SCID mice passively immunised with rabbit polyclonal antiserum to recombinant SREHP/trpE were protected against an intrahepatic challenged with virulent *E. histolytica* HM1 : IMSS trophozoites. Because this study was performed in SCID mice, which lack lymphocyte-based immunity, protection in this system was clearly antibody-mediated, providing some of the strongest evidence for a protective role of pre-existing anti-amebic antibodies in preventing the development of amebic liver abscess. It should also be emphasized that in these experiments, the ability of anti-amebic serum to inhibit amebic adherence correlated with protection from amebic liver abscess (10).

The efficacy of parenteral vaccination with SREHP was first tested in a gerbil model of amebic liver abscess (28). In these studies, recombinant SREHP as a maltose binding protein (MBP) fusion protein was used as the vaccine antigen. Recombinant SREHP was chosen for these studies because it could be more easily obtained in large quantities than native SREHP, it was better structurally defined (as it lacks the post-translational modifications of native SREHP) and it allowed for expression of different regions of the SREHP molecule. The SREHP cDNA had been expressed as trpE, glutathione-S-transferase (GST) maltose binding protein (MBP) fusion proteins in *Escherichia coli* (9, 29), and in baculovirus (21), but the highest yield of soluble protein was obtained with MBP as the fusion partner, hence this was the preparation used for the vaccine studies. The SREHP/MBP fusion protein contained most of the SREHP molecule, but lacked the signal sequence and the putative membrane-spanning domain of the C-terminus. In the initial study, gerbils, which develop amebic liver abscess after direct hepatic inoculation with *E. histolytica* trophozoites, were utilized. Gerbils received either three doses of SREHP/MBP intraperitoneally or a single dose intradermally, while control animals received the MBP protein by the identical route (28). Three weeks following vaccination, gerbils were challenged with an intrahepatic inoculation of amebic trophozoites, and 7 days later were sacrificed, and the size of any amebic liver abscess formed (expressed as the percentage of liver abscessed) measured. Among animals vaccinated with SREHP/MBP by the intraperitoneal route, 64% were protected from amebic liver abscess, while none of the gerbils vaccinated by the intradermal route showed abscess formation. All control animals developed amebic liver abscess in this study. Subsequently, a second trial of SREHP/MBP by the intraperitoneal route was performed, and this time it had 100% protective efficacy (30). How vaccination with SREHP/MBP provides protection against amebic liver abscess in gerbils has yet to be completely defined. Cell mediated immunity (as measured by delayed-type hypersensitivity) and antibody responses to both ameba and SREHP developed in SREHP/MBP vaccinated gerbils (28). The success of passive immunisation with anti-SREHP antibodies in SCID mice would suggest an important role for the induction of anti-SREHP antibodies in the protection seen, but there were no significant differences in the magnitude of the anti-SREHP or anti-amebic antibody response between the few vaccine failures (gerbils that received SREHP/ MBP but developed amebic liver abscess), and those vaccinated animals protected against disease (10, 28). However, whether there were differences in the epitopes recognised by the antibodies in protected animals compared to vaccine failures was not addressed in this study. This is probably critically important, for, as will be discussed below, a recent study looking at protection following vaccination with the 170 kDa subunit of the galactose-inhibitable lectin found significant differences in the epitopes recognised by animals protected by vaccination compared to those developing disease (31).

In a small trial, the safety and immunogenicity of the recombinant SREHP/MBP vaccine was tested in non-human primates (32). African Green Monkeys (n = 2) were vaccinated with SREHP/MBP and complete Freund's adjuvant in three doses at days 0, 30, and 53 by subcutaneous administration, while a control monkey received PBS and adjuvant alone at the same time points. Side effects from the SREHP/MBP vaccine consisted only of some local inflammation at the vaccination site, and this was not more extensive than that seen in the control monkey receiving adjuvant alone. The vaccinated monkeys developed anti-SREHP and anti-amebic antibodies following the first booster dose of SREHP/MBP, and titers did not significantly increase following the subsequent booster. No anti-amebic or anti-SREHP antibodies were detected in the control monkey. Since one of the goals of SREHP vaccination was to produce antibodies capable of blocking amebic adherence, this property was tested in the vaccinated monkeys. Serum from the SREHP/MBP vaccinated monkeys, obtained after the first or second booster immunisation, inhibited the adherence of *E. histolytica* trophozoites to Chinese Hamster Ovary (CHO) cells in vitro (32). Unfortunately, the protective efficacy of SREHP/MBP vaccination could not be tested in this study, as *E. histolytica*-naive (based on amebic serology and stool examination for amebic trophozoites) African Green Monkeys failed to develop amebic liver abscess even after direct hepatic inoculation with virulent *E. histolytica* trophozoites (32).

The success of parenteral immunisation with SREHP/MBP has led to attempts to stimulate mucosal immune responses to the SREHP molecule. This is based on the concept that a vaccine capable of stimulating mucosal IgA anti-amebic antibodies which block amebic adherence to intestinal epithelial cells could provide protection against both *E. histolytica* colonisation and disease. To date, the most widely used approach to inducing gut mucosal IgA responses has been oral immunisation. Oral vaccines have the potential to stimulate mucosal immune responses to a given adjuvant, and they have significant advantages as vaccines, because they are easier to administer, may have lower costs, and are preferred to injection by many vaccine recipients. The fundamental problem with oral vaccines has been how to make orally administered antigens immunogenic. Most antigens are not naturally immunogenic when administered by the oral route, hence the use of specific adjuvants and specialized delivery modes have become critical in oral vaccine development. In the case of SREHP, two major approaches have been used. The first approach is based on the oral administration of SREHP, or peptides derived from SREHP, in conjunction with the non-toxic B subunit of cholera toxin. The second approach has been centered on the expression and delivery of the recombinant SREHP molecule by attenuated *Salmonella* or *Vibrio cholerae* carriers.

The rationale for combining SREHP with the cholera toxin B subunit (CtxB) for oral immunisation derived from the recognised mucosal adjuvant properties of cholera toxin (CT). The structure of CT has been solved by X-ray crystallography, and is known to consist of one A subunit, which contains the active toxin domain (A1), as well as a short sequence (A2), which serves to link the A subunit non-covalently to five B subunits (33). The five B subunits each bind to a single molecule of G_{M1} ganglioside on the surface of intestinal cells, and this allows the internalization of the A subunit into the intestinal epithelial cells with resultant intoxication (34). When administered orally, CT induces high levels of mucosal IgA and serum IgA anti-toxin antibodies, as well as serum IgG anti-toxin antibodies in animals (35). CT is also one of the few molecules that can serve as a mucosal adjuvant. When a complex protein, such as keyhole limpet hemocyanin (KLH), is administered orally, it normally does not induce the production of mucosal or serum anti-KLH antibodies. However, when KLH is administered in conjunction with CT by the oral route, both anti-CT and anti-KLH mucosal and serum antibodies are produced (35–37). The mechanism underlying the adjuvant properties of CT has been controversial, and questions have arisen as to whether the toxin activity of the molecule is required for adjuvant activity, and whether the non-toxic B subunit alone has adjuvant activity (38–47). In two recent studies, investigators designed mutant CT molecules and were able to dissociate the diarrheagenic properties of the molecule from its adjuvant effects (as measured by the immune response to intranasal administration of proteins with the mutant molecules) (48, 49). There is also evidence to suggest that there may be interspecies differences in the CtxB response, as the B subunit alone may serve as an effective adjuvant in humans, but not in mice (50, 51).

One potential mechanism by which CtxB could facilitate the immune response to an antigen is by its targeting function to host G_{M1} ganglioside. By fusing a molecule to CtxB one could potentially deliver it to intestinal epithelial cells expressing G_{M1} ganglioside on their surface, and in turn, increase the opportunity for its (the antigen) internalisation and presentation to lymphocytes. This approach was the basis for the development of genetic constructs which allow the fusion of peptides to the CtxB protein (52, 53). These constructs were used to engineer a fusion protein (CtxB : SREHP-12) that contains the dodecapeptide repeat of SREHP fused to CtxB (54). The CtxB:SREHP-12 protein was expressed in *E. coli*, and could be purified by a two-step procedure. Critically, the CtxB moiety in the chimeric protein maintained the ability to bind to G_{M1} ganglioside, as the CtxB : SREHP-12 fusion protein was as potent as CtxB alone in blocking the binding of labeled CtxB to G_{M1} ganglioside (54). To test the immunogenicity of the CtxB : SREHP-12 fusion protein, mice received 4 oral doses at weekly intervals of CtxB : SREHP-12 and a subclinical dose of CT. Control mice were orally vaccinated with CtxB alone, and the subclinical dose of cholera toxin with the same schedule. Mice vaccinated with CtxB : SREHP-12 produced IgA anti-amebic antibodies in stool and bile, and had significant numbers of antibody-secreting cells producing anti-SREHP and anti-amebic antibodies in mesenteric lymph nodes and spleen (54). Mice orally vaccinated with CtxB did not develop anti-SREHP or anti-amebic antibodies and the number of antibody secreting cells recognising SREHP or *E. histolytica* trophozoites in control mice did not differ from background levels in any assay. CtxB and CtxB : SREHP-12 vaccinated mice produced anti-CtxB antibodies demonstrating that the linkage of SREHP to the CtxB protein did not significantly alter the immunogenicity of CtxB (54). One limitation of this study was the use of a subclinical dose of CT in addition to the CtxB : SREHP-12 fusion protein, which was employed because of concerns about the adjuvant effects of CtxB alone in mice (54). In a recent study, the CtxB : SREHP-12 molecule was administered to mice without the subclinical dose of CT, and still proved effective in generating a mucosal immune response to *E. histolytica* (55). These studies established CtxB : SREHP-12 as one of the first candidates for a oral vaccine to prevent amebiasis.

The CtxB : SREHP-12 protein, while effective, only utilised a portion of the SREHP molecule as the vaccine antigen. To create a vaccine that contains all of the SREHP sequence (with the exception of the signal sequence and putative membrane-spanning domain) linked to CtxB, a strategy that utilises fusion of SREHP to the A2 peptide of CT was used (56). It has been previously shown that antigens, such as maltose binding protein (MBP) can be fused to the A2 (the CtxB-binding portion) segment of the cholera toxin A moiety (56). When these molecules are co-expressed in *E. coli* with CtxB, a "pseudotoxin" molecule is formed, where the antigen of interest, rather than the toxic CtxA domain, is linked to the CtxB subunits (56). Recently, SREHP/ MBP was fused to CtxA2, and a holotoxin-like molecule consisting of SREHP/ MBP complexed to CtxB (SREHP-H) was created (55) Mice orally vaccinated with SREHP-H developed mucosal IgA and serum IgG anti-amebic antibody responses. A comparison between oral SREHP-H and CtxB : SREHP-12 immunisation revealed slightly higher levels of anti-amebic antibodies in SREHP-H vaccinated mice, but this difference was not statistically significant (55). Taken as a whole, these studies indicate that coupling the SREHP molecule, (or one of its dodecapeptide repeats) to CtxB creates a fusion protein that is mucosally immunogenic, inducing anti-amebic antibodies in mice and gerbils. While these strategies are very promising, the recent development of mutant CT molecules that are "non-toxic" but retain adjuvant activity appears to offer an important advance in this field, and these molecules may become the preferred adjuvants for inducing mucosal antibody responses (48, 49). It also should be emphasised that it has yet to be shown that the mucosal anti-amebic antibodies created after immunisation can protect animals against intestinal amebiasis.

One of the strategies currently being used in the design of vaccines to prevent amebiasis is the delivery of amebic antigens to the host by oral immunisation with attenuated vaccine strains of *Salmonella* species or *Vibrio cholerae* that express recombinant *E. histolytica* proteins. This approach has the obvious advantage of potentially inducing protective mucosal immune responses to two diseases with one vaccine. *Salmonella* spp. are desirable vectors to deliver amebic antigens because oral vaccination with salmonellae expressing heterologous antigens can induce mucosal IgA, as well as serum IgG and cell-mediated immune responses to the foreign antigens (57). While the gut mucosal IgA response may provide a first line of defense against *E. histolytica*, if amebic trophozoites invade through colonic mucosal layers, serum antibody or cell-mediated immune responses may become much more important in host defense than mucosal IgA.

The SREHP/MBP fusion protein has been successfully expressed in attenuated vaccine strains of salmonellae that have engineered deletions in cAMP receptor (*crp*), and adenyl cyclase (*cya*) encoding genes (58–60). These strains also have an engineered deletion in the *asd* gene which results in a requirement for diaminopilmelic acid (DAP) for bacterial growth (61). Provision of the *asd* gene within a plasmid which also contained the SREHP/MBP gene, provided a non-antibiotic resistance selectable marker for transformation (59, 61). The ability to avoid antibiotic resistance markers is extremely desirable in bacterial strains destined for human or animal vaccine use. Mice vaccinated in a three dose oral schedule with *S. typhimurium* χ4550 (Δ*cya*Δ*crp*Δ*asd*) expressing SREHP/MBP produced mucosal IgA anti-amebic antibodies in their saliva and stool, and IgG anti-amebic antibodies in their serum (60). Mice vaccinated with the *S. typhimurium*/SREHP vaccine also produced mucosal and serum antibodies to *S. typhimurium* LPS, indicating that expression of the SREHP/MBP molecule did not alter the immunogenicity of the *S. typhimurium* carrier (60). The success of the *S. typhimurium*/SREHP vaccine in inducing serum IgG anti-amebic antibodies led to a study of whether this vaccine could provide protection against amebic liver abscess. Gerbils vaccinated with *S. typhimurium*/SREHP developed mucosal IgA anti-amebic antibodies in stool and IgG anti-amebic antibodies in serum. Strikingly, 78% of *S. typhimurium*/SREHP vaccinated gerbils were completely protected against the development of ALA, while no protection against amebic liver abscess was seen in gerbils vaccinated with attenuated *S. typhimurium* expressing a control plasmid (60).

These experiments demonstrated that *S. typhimurium* can serve as an effective delivery system for the amebic SREHP molecule, and showed that vaccination by the oral route can provide protection against amebic liver abscess. For a vaccine designed for human use, attenuated *S. typhi* strains represent a more desirable carrier for amebic antigens than *S. typhimurium*, as they provide for the possibility of a combination amebiasis/typhoid fever vaccine. The SREHP/MBP fusion protein has been successfully expressed in *S. typhi* TY2 χ4297 (Δ*cya*Δ*crp*Δ*asd*), an attenuated vaccine strain of *S. typhi* (62). While the mucosal immunity of the *S. typhi* TY2 χ4297/SREHP strain could not be assessed in mice (because of the host specificity of *S. typhi*), the SREHP molecule remained immunogenic, as mice parenterally immunized with *S. typhi* TY2 χ4297 (Δ*cya*Δ*crp*Δ*asd*) expressing SREHP/MBP developed serum anti-amebic antibodies (62). Importantly, expression of the SREHP/

MBP fusion protein did not alter the attenuation of the *S. typhi* vaccine strain based on its LD50 in mice. The *S. typhi* TY2 χ4297 strain has been previously tested in humans, making the *S. typhi* TY2 χ4297/SREHP vaccine a candidate for testing in phase I human trials (63).

An alternative approach for delivering SREHP which preserves the concept of a dual purpose vaccine has been the expression of CtxB : SREHP-12 in an attenuated strain of *V. cholerae* (64). The CtxB : SREHP-12 coding sequence was inserted into the live El Tor *Vibrio cholerae* vaccine strain Peru2 at a chromosomal insertion site [Peru2(ETR3)] or was expressed on a plasmid [Peru2(pETR5.1)]. Both strains proved immunogenic, as neonatal mice orally vaccinated with either Peru2(ETR3) or Peru2(pETR5.1) developed anti-amebic and vibriocidal antibodies. However, the levels of serum and mucosal anti-amebic antibodies were higher in mice receiving the Peru2(pETR5.1) vaccine, probably reflecting higher levels of CtxB : SREHP-12 expression in the Peru2(pETR5.1) vaccine strain (64). These results suggest that *V. cholerae* strains expressing SREHP can be successful oral delivery systems for the induction of mucosal and systemic anti-amebic and anti-*V. cholerae* immune responses.

The *E. histolytica* Galactose-Inhibitable Lectin

One of the leading vaccine candidates for amebiasis is the galactose-inhibitable lectin. The structure of this molecule, and its multiple functions have been discussed in detail in chapters 4 and 5, and will not be reviewed extensively here. A number of the properties of the lectin would appear to make it an excellent candidate antigen for an amebiasis vaccine. The galactose-inhibitable lectin appears to play an important role in amebic binding to mammalian cells, and monoclonal antibodies directed against certain regions of the lectin can inhibit amebic adherence to CHO cells (8). Interestingly, it was also found that monoclonal antibodies to other epitopes of the molecule can actually enhance the adherence of *E. histolytica* trophozoites to CHO cells, indicating that selection of the proper epitopes could be crucial in developing an effective vaccine using the galactose-inhibitable lectin (65). An anti-amebic monoclonal antibody that renders *E. histolytica* trophozoites susceptible to killing by human complement components C5b9 was found to bind epitopes within the cysteine-rich region of the 170-kDa subunit of the galactose-inhibitable lectin, suggesting that the lectin could play a role in the ability of *E. histolytica* trophozoites to resist killing by human complement (66). This suggests that a vaccine that produced complement sensitivity in *E. histolytica* by inducing antibodies to this region of the 170 kDa subunit of the lectin could be very effective in preventing the establishment of extra-intestinal amebiasis.

More than 90% of patients with amebic liver abscess develop antibodies capable of binding to the native galactose-inhibitable lectin, and essentially all of these antibodies appear to be directed against the 170-kDa subunit (67). The derived amino acid sequence of the 170 kDa subunit of the lectin has been used to demarcate 3 structural domains of the molecule, a cysteine-poor region, a pseudorepeat region, and a cysteine-rich region. In one study, recombinant fusion proteins containing each of the domains linked to glutathione-S-transferase (GST) were screened with antibodies from patients in several different geographic regions with ALA (68). All individuals screened had antibodies to the entire 170-kDa molecule and to the cysteine-rich region (170CR fusion protein), most had antibodies to the cysteine-poor domain of the molecule (170CP fusion protein), but few had antibodies that bound to the pseudorepeat region (68). The immunogenic properties of the cysteine-rich region of the 170-kDa subunit have been confirmed and extended by studies showing that more than 95% of sera from patients with amebic liver abscess have serum IgA antibodies that recognize a recombinant protein derived from the cysteine-rich domain of the 170-kDa subunit (69), and more than 80% of individuals with amebic colitis develop mucosal IgA antibodies that bind this recombinant protein (70).

The purified native galactose-inhibitable lectin was the first defined *E. histolytica* antigen tested as an amebiasis vaccine (3). Gerbils vaccinated with the purified lectin developed antibodies against the 170-kDa subunit of the molecule; antibodies to the light subunit were not detected. Serum from vaccinated gerbils blocked amebic adherence to CHO cells when used at a 1/10 dilution, but enhanced adherence when used at a 1/1,000 dilution. Vaccination with the purified galactose-inhibitable lectin was protective, as only 27% of vaccinated gerbils developed an amebic liver abscess compared with 81% of control animals which received only the adjuvant (3). An analysis of the size of the amebic liver abscess in vaccinated animals revealed that the amebic liver abscesses detected in gerbils vaccinated with the galactose-inhibitable lectin were significantly larger than those seen in the adjuvant control gerbils, suggesting that some component of the immune response to vaccination with the native lectin could exacerbate disease in a subgroup of gerbils. This study was the first to demonstrate that vaccination with a purified amebic antigen could provide protection against amebic liver abscess, and clearly established the potential of the galactose-inhibitable lectin as a candidate vaccine antigen.

Subsequent studies have looked at recombinant antigens derived from the sequence of the galactose-inhibitable lectin as vaccines to prevent amebic liver abscess. The use of recombinant antigens was felt to be particularly valuable for the galactose-inhibitable lectin, because one could easily use only the heavy subunit of the lectin, and even specific domains of that molecule. This might favor the development of a recombinant galactose-inhibitable lectin based vaccine that could mimic the protective effects of the native molecule without any exacerbating effects on amebic liver abscess. Initial studies employed recombinant proteins containing the cysteine-rich domain of the 170CR subunit (30, 69). Among gerbils vaccinated with a recombinant antigen containing amino acids 649 to 1202 of the 170-kDa subunit of the galactose-inhibitable lectin fused to glutathione-S-transferase (GST) in Freund's adjuvant, only 17% developed an amebic liver abscess compared with 100% of PBS/adjuvant-vaccinated gerbils and 90% of GST/adjuvant-vaccinated gerbils (30). This level of protection was equivalent or superior to vaccination with the native galactose-inhibitable lectin, and the few vaccine "failures" in this study, i.e. gerbils that were vaccinated with the 170CR protein but did develop an amebic liver abscess, did not have abscesses that were larger than either the GST-vaccinated or PBS-vaccinated control groups (3, 30). In an independent study, the protective efficacy of a different recombinant protein derived from the cysteine-rich region of the lectin was studied in gerbils (69). The recombinant protein, designated LC3, contained amino acids 758 to 1134 of the 170-kDa subunit of the galactose-inhibitable lectin fused to six histidine residues. Among gerbils vaccinated with the fusion protein (designated LC3) and the adjuvant Titermax, only 19% developed an amebic liver abscess after direct hepatic inoculation with *E. histolytica* trophozoites, compared with 59% of gerbils receiving Titermax alone, for a vaccine protective efficacy of 68%. In this study as well, the size of the amebic liver abscess in recombinant vaccine failures was not significantly larger than that seen in control animals (69). Taken together, these studies indicated that recombinant antigen vaccines based on sequences from the cysteine-rich region of the galactose-inhibitable lectin could match the efficacy of vaccination with the native molecule in preventing amebic liver abscess in gerbils, and lacked the potential exacerbating effects seen with the native molecule (3, 30, 69).

A recent study has further defined the protective and exacerbating responses to vaccination with the 170 kDa subunit of the lectin. Recombinant proteins (as non-fusion proteins) corresponding to four domains of the lectin, two domains within the cysteine rich region (CR1 and CR2), the pseudorepeat region (PR) and the cysteine-poor region (CP), as well as synthetic peptides derived from specific regions of each of these domains were synthesised, than used to (1) immunise gerbils to assess protection from amebic liver abscess; (2) immunise rabbits, whose serum was used for passive immunisation studies in the SCID mouse model of amebic liver abscess; (3) be target antigens in Western blotting studies using serum from individuals with amebiasis (31). It was found that protective immunity after vaccination could be correlated with the development of an antibody response to a region of 25 amino acids located in the CR2 domain of the molecule. Gerbils vaccinated with the recombinant protein containing this region, and SCID mice passively immunized with rabbit antibodies against this 25 amino acid region showed high levels of protection against amebic liver abscess. The potential clinical relevance of this finding was demonstrated in immunoblotting studies using serum from patients with amebiasis. Strikingly, individuals who were colonised with *E. histolytica*, but had no evidence of invasive disease, had a high prevalence of antibodies to the protective domain, while individuals who presented with amebic colitis or amebic liver abscess did not possess antibodies to this region of the galactose-inhibitable lectin (31).

The fine specificity of the antibody response to the 170 kDa subunit of the galactose-inhibitable lectin also determines whether prior vaccination actually exacerbates disease when gerbils are challenged with ameba. Gerbils vaccinated with the recombinant protein containing only the CP domain of the 170 kDa subunit of the lectin developed significantly larger amebic liver abscesses than gerbils receiving adjuvant alone. Evidence that this effect is antibody-mediated came from the passive immunization studies in SCID mice, where amebic liver abscess were significantly larger in mice receiving antiserum to the CP region, than in mice receiving pre-immune antiserum (31). Taken as a whole, the results of this study provide critical information for designing amebiasis vaccines based on the 170 kDa subunit of the galactose-inhibitable lectin, and represent the strongest evidence to date that it is the antibody response that mediates protective immunity to amebiasis. It is worth emphasising that it appears to be the fine-specificity of that antibody response, not its magnitude, that determines whether protection is achieved.

Several approaches have been used to produce gut mucosal antibodies to the 170 kDa subunit of the galactose-inhibitable lectin. In one study, rats were immunised with the purified native lectin and Freund's adjuvant parenterally, than received an intra-Peyer's Patch injection of the purified lectin with either incomplete Freund's adjuvant or CtxB (5). Anti-lectin sIgA responses were significantly higher in those animals receiving CtxB, and sIgA obtained from these animals could block the adherence of *E. histolytica* trophozoites to mammalian cells.

This study indicated that mucosal antibodies capable of blocking amebic adherence could be generated by immunisation with the native galactose-inhibitable adhesin. Subsequently, it was shown that oral immunisation of mice with the recombinant LC3 protein (containing amino acids 758 to 1134 of the 170 kDa subunit) and cholera toxin can generate secretory IgA antibodies against the LC3 protein (71) Importantly, intestinal secretions obtained from mice orally immunised with LC3/cholera toxin could block the adherence of amebic trophozoites to Chinese Hamster Ovary cells, establishing for the first time that oral vaccination with a recombinant amebic antigen can induce adherence-blocking antibodies in animals (71).

Oral immunisation with attenuated Salmonella expressing a portion of the 170 kDa subunit of the galactose-inhibitable lectin has recently been described (72). Attenuated strains of *S. dublin* and *S. typhimurium* were transformed with plasmids containing the coding region for amino acids 482-1138 or amino acids 2 to 596 of the lectin fused to the GST gene. Expression of the fusion protein by the *Salmonella* strains was achieved, but gerbils orally vaccinated with either construct failed to develop detectable serum anti-lectin antibodies. Mucosal immune responses were not assayed in this study. Despite the lack of an antibody response, gerbils vaccinated with *Salmonella* expressing the galactose-inhibitable lectin/GST fusion protein had smaller amebic liver abscesses after direct hepatic inoculation of amebic trophoziotes than those gerbils receiving control strains of *Salmonella* (72). The finding of smaller abscesses suggests some form of protection is occurring, but it is unclear from the study whether smaller abscesses reflect a healing of established lesions, or simply a delay in abscess formation. These results differ from those seen with vaccination with *S. typhimurium* expressing SREHP/MBP, where high levels of anti-amebic antibodies were seen in vaccinated gerbils, and complete protection from amebic liver abscess was seen in most animals (60). The difference between these studies may not relate to differences in the immunogenicity or protective efficacy between the two amebic antigens, but rather may reflect differences in the level of expression of the recombinant proteins, and the duration of recombinant protein expression once the bacteria is in the host animal (60, 72). In the case of SREHP/MBP expression in *S. typhimurium* χ4550 ($\Delta cya\,\Delta crp\,\Delta asd$), the use of a high-copy number plasmid which clearly increased SREHP/MBP expression, and the presence of constant selective pressure for the *asd*-containing plasmid which insures that bacteria continue to express SREHP/MBP even within the host, may have led to a more effective vaccine (60). Given the protective efficacy of the 170 kDa antigen in parenteral studies, it seems likely that improvements in the oral delivery system would improve the immunogenicity and protective efficacy of oral vaccination with this molecule.

Other Candidate Antigens for an Amebiasis Vaccine

One of the better studied candidate vaccine antigens has been a 29-kDa cysteine-rich amebic antigen that was first identified by anti-amebic antibody screening of an *E. histolytica* cDNA library (73). The derived amino acid sequence of a full length cDNA and genomic clones showed that the 29-kDa protein has significant relatedness to the sequences of hydrogen peroxide inactivating proteins that are found in gut-living prokaryotes (74). Where the 29 kDa molecule is actually located in amebic trophozoites has been the subject of controversy. The putative function of this molecule, the absence of a signal sequence, and indirect immunofluorescence studies suggest that the 29-kDa antigen is located in the cytoplasm and nucleus of *E. histolytica* trophozoites (74, 75). However, surface labeling studies, indirect immuno-fluorescence, and transmission electron microscopy with immunogold support a surface membrane location for the 29-kDa antigen (73, 76, 77). Regardless of its location, the 29-kDa molecule is immunogenic. Among individuals with amebic liver abscess, roughly 80% develop antibodies that bind to the native or recombinant 29-kDa protein (78, 79). Vaccine studies with the 29 kDa antigen have used a recombinant protein derived from the sequence of a full length cDNA clone fused to sequences encoding six histidine residues (79). Gerbils immunized with the recombinant 29-kDa fusion protein produced antibodies that recognized the native 29-kDa protein in amebic lysates, while sera from control gerbils showed no reactivity with the native molecule. Vaccination with the recombinant 29-kDa protein provided gerbils with some protection against amebic liver abscess after direct hepatic challenge with *E. histolytica* trophozoites. Approximately 30% of gerbils vaccinated with the recombinant 29-kDa protein, developed an amebic liver abscess, compared to 59% of gerbils in the adjuvant control group, giving a calculated vaccine efficacy of 49% (79).

There are a number of other *E. histolytica* antigens that represent potential candidates for inclusion in an amebiasis vaccine. *E. histolytica* possesses a family of neutral cysteine proteinases that are recognized virulence factors, and appear to play a critical role in amebic invasion and destruction of host extracellular matrix tissues (80–82). Neutralisation of the effects of cysteine proteinase by proteinase inhibitors, or by administration of laminin, can reduce the size of amebic liver abscess in SCID mice (83, 84). The proteinases appear to be naturally immunogenic, as patients who have had amebic liver abscess make antibodies that recognise amebic cysteine proteinase (85). Another potential vaccine candidates are the family of amebapores, pore-forming peptides that play a critical role in the cytolytic activity of *E. histolytica* trophozoites (86). If immunisation with amebapores, or isoforms of the molecules that lack cytolytic activity, can generate neutralising antibodies capable of blocking the cytolytic effects of amebapore, it might provide an effective anti-disease vaccine (87–89). Other vaccine candidates include the 96-kDa *E. histolytica* alcohol dehydrogenase 2 (EhADH2), which possesses both alcohol dehydrogenase and acetaldehyde dehydrogenase activity, and plays a key role in the amebic fermentation pathway (90, 91). While most of the 96 kDa protein is probably located within the cytoplasm, at least some of the EhADH2 enzyme or an isoform can be detected on the surface of amebic trophozoites. Studies of the EhADH2 molecule indicate that it can bind to extracellular matrix proteins such as fibronectin and laminin, suggesting it could have functions other than its key role in fermentation (90). A recombinant version of the EhADH2 protein which maintains enzyme activity and the ability to bind to extracellular matrix proteins has been produced in *E. coli* and did not require a fusion partner (92).

The amebic glycoconjugate is a highly abundant surface molecule that contains phosphate, sugars, and is linked to the membrane by a GPI anchor (93). While these features are reminiscent of those seen with Leishmania lipophosphoglycan (LPG) molecules, detailed structural data on the amebic glycoconjugate is not yet available. The glycoconjugate is highly immunogenic, and antibodies to this molecule block amebic adherence to mammalian cells (93). Recently, it was shown that SCID mice passively immunised with a monoclonal antibody to the amebic glycoconjugate are protected against developing amebic liver abscess after direct hepatic challenge with amebic trophozoites (94). While these data are promising, more structural information, and the identification of the protective epitopes will probably be necessary before this becomes a viable vaccine candidate.

Combination Vaccines for Amebiasis

Vaccines that utilise multiple recombinant amebic antigens might prove more effective than single antigen vaccines. For example, individuals who do not develop a response to one antigen, might develop a protective response to the other component of the vaccine. Alternatively, the immune response to both antigens might provide better protective efficacy than the response to a single antigen (e.g. synergistic effects of anti-adherence antibodies directed against two different targets). In one study, gerbils were parenterally vaccinated with a combination of recombinant proteins derived from the SREHP molecule and the 170 kDa subunit of the galactose-inhibitable lectin (30). Gerbils receiving both the SREHP/MBP and 170CR/GST vaccines developed antibodies that recognized both the native 170 kDa subunit of the galactose-inhibitable adhesin, and the SREHP molecule. Vaccinated gerbils were protected against amebic liver abscess, with 14% of SREHP/MBP and 170CR/GST vaccinated gerbils developing amebic liver abscess compared to 100% and 90% of MBP and GST-vaccinated gerbils respectively (30). While these results indicate that the combination vaccine was highly effective in preventing amebic liver abscess in gerbils, when the results were compared to those obtained with vaccination with SREHP/MBP alone or vaccination with 170CR/GST alone, they did not reveal an advantage in protective efficacy for the combination vaccine. However, these data do demonstrate that simultaneous administration of the SREHP/MBP and 170CR vaccines does not appear to diminish the immune response to either antigen, and suggest that a combination vaccine containing those two antigens is feasible.

Problems in Amebiasis Vaccine Development

The studies cited above have demonstrated the feasibility of developing recombinant antigen-based vaccines to prevent amebic liver abscess, and shown that *E. histolytica* antigens can be delivered via the oral route to stimulate mucosal immune responses to ameba. While these results are encouraging, there are some important limitations to these studies that need to be addressed. To date, all studies of the efficacy of vaccination in providing protection against amebic liver abscess have been performed in a single animal model, the gerbil, and use an artificial form of establishing amebic liver abscess, direct hepatic inoculation of trophozoites. While direct inoculation may actually represent a more stringent challenge than the natural mechanism of amebic liver abscess formation in humans (i.e. hematogenous spread via the portal vein of what is probably significantly fewer amebae into the liver), the predictive value of the gerbil model for humans is unknown. Another important question is the duration of protective immunity in vaccinated animals. In essentially all studies, vaccinated animals have been challenged at time points (1 to 3 weeks following booster immunisations) when circulating anti-amebic antibodies are detectable; whether protection would be seen at much later time points (e.g. 6 months) after vaccination needs to be studied. Another problem with current vaccine studies is the failure to incorporate challenge with "wild-type" *E. histolytica* into experiments. The cDNA sequences for the recombinant antigens used in these studies are generally derived from the HM1 : IMSS laboratory strain of *E. histolytica*, which is the same strain used as the challenge organism in all studies. Although there is abundant serologic evidence indicating that there are highly conserved epitopes in the SREHP, 170-kDa galactose-inhibitable lectin, and 29-kDa antigens (24, 67–69, 78, 79), the efficacy of these HM1 : IMSS-derived recombinant antigens as vaccines against clinical isolates of *E. histolytica* has not been established.

An important problem in assessing the efficacy of oral vaccines remains the lack of a good animal model for intestinal amebiasis. How one selects the best oral vaccine candidates for testing in humans in the absence of efficacy testing in animal models remains a difficult question. Another problem may lie in the potential delivery vectors for oral vaccines. While it is clear that mice orally vaccinated with *S. typhimurium* can develop immune responses to heterologous antigens expressed in these vaccine strains, it less clear that humans vaccinated with *S. typhi* expressing heterologous antigens will develop high level immune responses to the foreign antigen. In a recent study, female adult volunteers vaccinated with *S. typhi* TY2 χ4632 (Δ*cya* Δ*crp-cdt* Δ*asd*) expressing the pre-S1 protein of the hepatitis B virus developed anti-LPS antibodies but only one individual showed seroconversion to the pre-S1 protein (95). The same protein had been immunogenic when expressed by *S. typhimurium* and administered to mice (96). While these findings by no means invalidate this strategy, they do suggest that further developments may be necessary before *S. typhi* can be used as a carrier to induce consistent immune responses to heterologous antigens in humans.

Future Directions

The past decade has seen significant progress in attempts to develop a vaccine for amebiasis, but much work remains to be done. One of the first steps will be the testing of current vaccine constructs in humans. A number of candidate recombinant antigens have now been identified, and phase I trials need to be initiated to begin the process of testing their safety in humans. The recent progress in diagnosing *E. histolytica* infection and distinguishing it from *E. dispar* infection, the development of molecular epidemiologic tools, and important ongoing studies of the natural history of disease should provide the methods and information necessary for characterising large populations for vaccine efficacy trials. Even as current vaccine candidates are tested, an important area for further development will be improving the mode of delivery of antigens to stimulate mucosal immune responses. The recognition that intranasal immunisation may increase the mucosal immunogenicity of antigens, and the recent development of mutant cholera toxin molecules that retain adjuvant activity but do not cause diarrhea may provide powerful new tools towards the design of oral vaccines to prevent amebiasis. The push towards the development of food-based vaccines, with the expression of recombinant antigens in food plants, may represent another avenue for amebiasis vaccine development. Genetic (DNA) vaccines are being tested for several infectious diseases, and may provide a viable approach for an amebiasis vaccine. Finally, a continued commitment to amebiasis vaccine development, from scientists, physicians in endemic areas, and funding agencies will be necessary to realize the promise of an amebiasis vaccine.

Acknowledgments

I wish to acknowledge the many contributions of Tonghai Zhang to our efforts on vaccine development, and the financial support of NIH grants AI30084 and AI-01231, and WHO grant GPV-I5181281.

References

1. Caballero-Salcedo A, *et al.* (1994). *Am. J. Trop. Med. Hyg.* **4**: 412.
2. deLeon A (1970). *Arch. Invest. Med. De Mex.* **1**: s205.
3. Petri Jr WA and Ravdin JI (1990). *Infect. Immun.* **59**: 97.
4. Carrero JC, *et al.* (1994). *Infect. Immun.* **62**: 764.

5. Kelsall BL and Ravdin JI (1995). *Infect. Immun.* **63**: 686.
6. Ghosh PK, *et al.* (1994). *Arch. Med. Res.* **23**: 297.
7. Seydel KB, *et al.* (1997). *Infect. Immun.* **65**: 1631.
8. Ravdin JI, *et al.* (1986). *Infect. Immun.* **53**: 1.
9. Stanley Jr SL, *et al.* (1990). *Proc. Natl. Acad. Sci. USA* **87**: 4976.
10. Zhang T, *et al.* (1994). *Parasite Immunol.* **16**: 225.
11. Swartzwelder JC and Avant WH (1952). *Am. J. Trop. Med. Hyg.* **1**: 567.
12. Vazquez-Saavedra JA, *et al.* (1973). *Arch. Invest. Med. De Mex.* **Suppl 1**: 15.
13. Jain P, *et al.* (1980). *Trans. R. Soc. Trop. Med. Hyg.* **74**: 347.
14. Clark CG (1995). *J. Eukaryot. Microbiol.* **42**: 590.
15. Navarro-García F, *et al.* (1997). *Clin. Immunol. Immunopathol.* **82**: 221.
16. Swartzwelder JC and Muller GR (1950). *Am. J. Trop. Med. Hyg.* **30**: 181.
17. Ghadirian E and Meerovitch E (1978). *J. Parasitol.* **64**: 742.
18. Ghadirian E, *et al.* (1980). *Am. J. Trop. Med. Hyg.* **29**: 779.
19. Jiminez-Cardoso JM, *et al.* (1989). *Rev. Invest. Clin. (Mex.)* **41**: 133.
20. Sharma A, *et al.* (1985). *Infect. Immun.* **48**: 634.
21. Stanley Jr SL, *et al.* (1995). *J. Biol. Chem.* **270**: 4121.
22. Köhler S and Tannich E (1993). *Mol. Biochem. Parasitol.* **59**: 49.
23. Samuelson J (1997). Personal communication.
24. Stanley Jr SL, *et al.* (1991). *JAMA* **266**: 1984.
25. Wang L, *et al.* (1997). *Am. J. Trop. Med. Hyg.* In press.
26. Li E, *et al.* (1992). *Mol. Biochem. Parasitol.* **50**: 355.
27. Clark CG and Diamond LS (1993). *Exp. Parasitol.* **77**: 450.
28. Zhang T, *et al.* (1994). *Infect. Immun.* **62**: 1166.
29. Myung K, *et al.* (1992). *Arch. Med. Res.* **23**: 285.
30. Zhang T and Stanley Jr SL (1994). *Infect. Immun.* **62**: 2605.
31. Lotter H, *et al.* (1997). *J. Exp. Med.* **185**: 1793.
32. Stanley Jr SL, *et al.* (1995). *Vaccine* **13**: 947.
33. Betley M, *et al.* (1989). *Annu. Rev. Microbiol.* **40**: 577.
34. Cuatrecasas P (1973). *Biochemistry* **12**: 3558.
35. Elson CO and Ealding W (1984). *J. Immunol.* **132**: 2736.
36. Elson CO and Ealding W (1984). *J. Immunol.* **133**: 2892.
37. Lycke N and Holmgren J (1986). *J. Immunol.* **59**: 301.
38. Russell MW and Wu H (1991). *Infect. Immun.* **59**: 4061.
39. McKenzie SJ and Halsey JF (1984). *J. Immunol.* **133**: 1818.
40. Bessen D and Fischetti V (1988). *Infect. Immun.* **56**: 2666.
41. Tamura S, *et al.* (1988). *Vaccine* **6**: 409.
42. Liang X, *et al.* (1988). *J. Immunol.* **141**: 1495.

43. Czerkinsky C, *et al.* (1989). *Infect. Immun.* **57**: 1072.
44. Dertzbaugh MT and Elson CO (1993). *Infect. Immun.* **61**: 48.
45. Lee A and Chen M (1994). *Infect. Immun.* **62**: 3594.
46. Gonzalez RA, *et al.* (1993). *Gene* **133**: 227.
47. Lycke N, *et al.* (1992). *Eur. J. Immunol.* **22**: 2277.
48. Douce G, *et al.* (1997). *Infect. Immun.* **65**: 2821.
49. Yamamoto S, *et al.* (1997). *Proc. Natl. Acad. Sci. USA* **94**: 5267.
50. Czerkinsky C, *et al.* (1993). *Clin. Infect. Dis.* **16 Suppl. 2**: S106.
51. Sanchez JL, *et al.* (1993). *J. Infect. Dis.* **167**: 1446.
52. Dertzbaugh MT, *et al.* (1990). *Infect. Immun.* **58**: 70.
53. Dertzbaugh MT and Macrina FL (1989). *Gene* **82**: 335.
54. Zhang T, *et al.* (1995). *Infect. Immun.* **63**: 1349.
55. Sultan F, *et al.* (1997). *Infect. Immun.* In press.
56. Jobling MG and Holmes RK (1992). *Infect. Immun.* **60**: 4915.
57. Curtiss RI, *et al.* (1989). *Cur. Top. Microb. Immunol.* **146**: 35.
58. Curtiss III R and Kelly SM (1987). *Infect. Immun.* **55**: 3035.
59. Cieslak PR, *et al.* (1993). *Vaccine* **11**: 773.
60. Zhang T and Stanley Jr SL (1996). *Infect. Immun.* **64**: 1526.
61. Nakayama K, *et al.* (1988). *Biotechnology* **6**: 693.
62. Zhang T and Stanley Jr SL (1997). *Vaccine.* In press.
63. Tacket CO, *et al.* (1992). *Infect. Immun.* **60**: 536.
64. Ryan ET, *et al.* (1997). *Infect. Immun.* **65**: 3118.
65. Petri Jr WA, *et al.* (1990). *J. Immunol.* **144**: 4803.
66. Braga LL, *et al.* (1992). *J. Clin. Invest.* **90**: 1131.
67. Ravdin JI, *et al.* (1990). *J. Infect. Dis.* **162**: 768.
68. Zhang Y, *et al.* (1992). *J. Clin. Microbiol.* **30**: 2788.
69. Soong C-JG, *et al.* (1995). *J. Infect. Dis.* **171**: 645.
70. Abou-El-Magd I, *et al.* (1996). *J. Infect. Dis.* **174**: 157.
71. Beving DE, *et al.* (1996). *Infect. Immun.* **64**: 1473.
72. Mann BJ, *et al.* (1997). *Vaccine* **15**: 659.
73. Torian BE, *et al.* (1990). *Proc. Natl. Acad. Sci. USA* **87**: 6358.
74. Bruchhaus I and Tannich E (1993). *Trop. Med. Parasitol.* **44**: 116.
75. Tachibana H, *et al.* (1990). *Infect. Immun.* **58**: 955.
76. Reed SL, *et al.* (1992). *Infect. Immun.* **60**: 542.
77. Flores BM, *et al.* (1993). *Mol. Microb.* **7**: 755.
78. Flores BM, *et al.* (1993). *J. Clin. Microbiol.* **31**: 1403.
79. Soong CG, *et al.* (1995). *Infect. Immun.* **63**: 472.
80. Tannich E, *et al.* (1991). *J. Biol. Chem.* **266**: 4798.
81. Keene WE, *et al.* (1990). *Exp. Parasitol.* **71**: 199.

82. Reed S, *et al* (1993). *J. Clin. Invest.* **91**: 1532.
83. Stanley Jr SL, *et al* (1995). *Infect. Immun.* **63**: 1587.
84. Li E, *et al.* (1995). *Infect. Immun.* **63**: 4150.
85. Osorio LM, *et al.* (1992). *Parasitology* **105**: 207.
86. Leippe M and Müller-Eberhard HJ (1994). *Toxicology* **87**: 5.
87. Leippe M, *et al.* (1994). *Proc. Natl. Acad. Sci. USA* **91**: 2602.
88. Andrä J, *et al.* (1996). *FEBS Lett.* **385**: 96.
89. Andrä J and Leippe M (1994). *FEBS Lett.* **354**: 97.
90. Yang W, *et al.* (1994). *Mol. Biochem. Parasitol.* **64**: 253.
91. Flores BM, *et al.* (1996). *J. Infect. Dis.* **173**: 226.
92. Yong T, *et al.* (1996). *Proc. Natl. Acad. Sci. USA* **93**: 6464.
93. Stanley Jr SL, *et al.* (1992). *Mol. Biochem. Parasitol.* **50**: 127.
94. Marinets A, *et al.* (1997) *J. Exp. Med.* In press.
95. Nardelli-Haefliger D, *et al.* (1996). *Infect. Immun.* **64**: 5219.
96. Schödel F, *et al.* (1994). *Infect. Immun.* **62**: 1669.

Chapter 8

Current Controversies

Jonathan I Ravdin, MD

Nesbitt Professor and Chair
Department of Medicine, University of Minnesota
420 Delaware Street, S.E., Minneapolis, MN 55455, USA
E-mail: ravdin001@gold.tc.umn.edu

Controversial issues in management of patients with amebiasis include whether to treat asymptomatic *Entamoeba* infection, how to best use serology and newer diagnostic tests, when to aspirate an amebic liver abscess, and what is the optimal, most efficacious, and least toxic therapy for amebic liver abscess. These issues are discussed, evidence is presented, and expert opinions are provided.

Effective management of patients with E. *histolytica* infection requires successful recognition of epidemiologic risk factors and the presentation of clinical amebiasis syndromes. The epidemiology of *Entamoeba* infection and the diagnosis and management of patients with colitis and extra-intestinal amebiasis are well presented in previous chapters. However, there are ambiguous or controversial areas that merit special attention and critical evaluation of the literature. Rarely are such issues discussed at length, due to a lack of consensus or availability of definitive clinical research studies.

Areas of controversy in clinical amebiasis (Table 1) include evaluation and treatment of people with asymptomatic intestinal infection, use of serology and newer diagnostic tests to replace microscopy of fecal samples, management of patients with amebic liver abscess, and use of luminal amebicides and other challenges in the treatment of invasive amebiasis.

Table 1. Controversies in clinical amebiasis.

- Should asymptomatic amebic infection be treated?
- Are there new quantitative diagnostic methods that can now replace microscopy of fecal samples?
- When is it necessary to aspirate an amebic liver abscess?
- When should luminal amebicides be used in treatment of amebiasis?

Asymptomatic Intestinal Infection

In this volume, David Mirelman provides a comprehensive review of the *in vitro* studies of *E dispar* and *E. histolytica*; Graham Clark and colleagues beautifully detailed the molecular differences of these two distinct species. However, until recently there have been no studies of asymptomatically infected individuals followed longitudinally over time nor any indication of whether natural immunity to intestinal infection occurs.

Saurgent and coworkers evaluated thousands of subjects worldwide with *E. dispar* intestinal infection; all were asymptomatic, never was an individual with disease found (1). Reports of abnormal intestinal pathology in such subjects were in uncontrolled studies in tropical areas where mucosal inflammation was as common in uninfected controls. Dr. Terry Jackson and I are conducting a large field study in Durban, South Africa, in which we are following over 1000 subjects prospectively every three weeks for up to 36 months. Asymptomatic *E. dispar* infection occurred commonly, with no evidence of disease nor systemic immune response.

In the light of all available evidence, individuals with asymptomatic *E. dispar* infection as confirmed by culture (2), antigen detection (3–4), or PCR (5–6) should not be treated. Infection is self-limited with spontaneous clearance over 6–12 months with no evidence of adverse effects (7–9). Importantly, serology for anti-amebic antibodies are negative (10). In endemic areas, re-infection with *E. dispar* is common and scarce public health resources should be dedicated elsewhere.

Determining how to manage asymptomatic *E. histolytica* infection is more complicated. Gathiram and Jackson (11) demonstrated that most subjects with intestinal infection by *E. histolytica* remain asymptomatic, despite development of a serum anti-amebic antibody response. In endemic areas of the tropical developing world, the standard of care is not to evaluate patients for asymptomatic intestinal parasitic infection (7). Patients with asymptomatic

Entamoeba infection are not treated, as methods to differentiate *dispar* from *histolytica* are unavailable in these settings. Serology for anti-amebic antibodies is less specific in endemic areas as up to 30% of uninfected controls have had prior *E. histolytica* infection and possess long-lived serum anti-amebic IgG antibodies (10). The duration after *E. histolytica* infection that serology tests positive is dependent on the method used, with agar gel diffusion or counterimmunoelectrophoresis becoming negative after approximately six months. Methods, such as ELISA or indirect hemagglutination, stay positive for up to ten years (9, 10). There is good evidence that the presence of hematophagous trophozoites (with ingested red blood cells) on fecal microscopy correlates highly with culture of *E. histolytica*, rather than *E. dispar*, from the stool (2). It is impossible at this time to predict which individuals or family members will go on to manifest invasive amebiasis when infected with *E. histolytica*. It seems prudent that, except under approved research protocols having close follow-up, patients determined to have asymptomatic *E. histolytica* infection should be treated with a luminal amebicide, such as diloxanide furoate (12, 13) or paramomycin (14, 15). Such circumstances are more likely to occur in developed world countries, in populations such as immigrants or travelers from endemic areas or in high-risk, chronically institutionalized populations.

Use of Serology and Newer Diagnostic Studies

Numerous studies have provided evidence that serology for anti-amebic antibodies, when intelligently applied, is an essential tool in diagnosing invasive amebiasis. Newer methodologies commercially available including ELISA, indirect hemoglutination, and agar gel diffusion. There is excellent data to indicate that after seven days of symptoms, over 85% of patients with invasive amebiasis have a positive serology for anti-amebic IgG antibodies (16–19). Therefore, in non-endemic areas, a positive test has a high positive predictive value (a true positive). This is more reliable than fecal microscopy, which has a high rate of error in developed world laboratories (20). Conversely, a negative serology after seven days of symptoms is strong evidence that an alternative diagnosis should be pursued. Serum anti-amebic IgM antibodies are found earlier in the clinical course (18), but IgM serology is not routinely available. In patients with less than seven days of symptoms, with appropriate epidemiologic risk factors, presentation, and a defect in the liver on ultrasound; negative serology (which should be repeated after a total of seven days of symptoms) should not at all affect the decision to treat. Patients with presumed inflammatory bowel disease should have an anti-amebic serology test before therapy with corticosteroids, especially if a biopsy has not been performed.

Fecal microscopy is relatively insensitive, as up to three separate tests are required to reach 90% sensitivity in patients with amebic colitis (21). In patients with amebic liver abscess, only 20% will be found to have *E. histolytica* in stool by microscopy; yet by culture, 72% will be positive (22). Clearly, more sensitive, specific, and quantitative diagnostic methodology is needed. Detection of amebic antigen in feces (3, 4, 17) and serum (3, 17, 18) by ELISA utilizing monoclonal and polyclonal anti-amebic antibodies has been studied, and at least two different kits are commercially available (4, 23). However, there is as yet insufficient clinical experience to assure their reliability and applicability; most laboratories do not have antigen detection tests available for *Entamoeba*. Recent studies are promising, demonstrating high sensitivity (compared to culture) and specificity for *dispar* or *histolytica*. Prospecture studies using seroconversion indicate that infection by *E. histolytica* is more common than by culture techniques. Our studies in South Africa, however, indicate that adverse field conditions such as lack of availability of refrigeration or access to rapid testing lead to decreased reliability. These factors could be solvable with further study and experimentation. PCR for detection of genomic DNA has greater sensitivity than antigen detection, but is not yet commercially available.

Management of Patients with Amebic Liver Abscess

Controversial areas in management of amebic liver abscess include the need for luminal amebicidal therapy, needle aspiration of abscesses, and chemotherapy with drugs such as chloroquine or emetine dehydrochloride. All patients should receive therapy with a nitro-imidazol, such as metronidazole or tinidazole, using various dosage regimes described by Sharon Reed in chapter 5. In addition, based on a recent study by Irusen and colleagues (22), all liver abscess patients should receive therapy with a luminal amebicide to avoid relapse due to persistent intestinal infection with *E. histolytica*. Most patients can be treated successfully without aspiration of the liver abscess (24–26) there is no evidence to indicate that routine aspiration results in a better outcome. Indications for aspiration (Table 2) include the need to rule out a bacterial abscess, prevention of rupture by

Table 2. Indications for aspiration of an amebic liver abscess.

- Failure to respond often three days to appropriate doses of nitroimidazol.
- High risk for bacterial (pyrogenic) liver abscess.
- Large abscesses (> 10 cm) with a thin rim of liver tissue.
- Left lobe abscesses abutting the liver capsule or pericardium.

---

a large abscess (> 10 cm) with a thin capsule of liver tissue, and lack of response to appropriate anti-amebic therapy within 72 hours. In addition, an abscess of the left lobe is more likely to rupture and should be aspirated if abutting the liver capsule or pericardium.

In some areas of the world, patients with amebic liver abscess are routinely treated with a combination of dehydroemetine and metronidazole. To my knowledge, despite extensive experience with use of this regimen, there is no controlled study indicating an improved outcome, as determined by clinical response and drug toxicity. Given the substantial cardiac toxicity of emetines and the fact that a metronidozole-resistant *E. histolytica* strain has never been observed, it seems prudent not to add emetine drugs or chloroquine to a nitroimidazole. As mentioned, failure to respond to metronidazole therapy is an indication for aspiration of the abscess.

Chemotherapy of Invasive Amebiasis

All patients should receive therapy with a luminal and tissue amebicidal agent. There is no clear data to indicate which luminal agent is preferred. Most authorities recommend diloxanide furoate as the drug of choice (12), but availability is limited (see chapter 5). Paramomycin (14, 15) and diiodohydroxyquin are alternative choices; although there are studies indicating that metronidazole, 750 mg, tid, for 10 days in adults will eradicate luminal infection, follow-up studies with culture were not performed. Amebic colitis has a worse prognosis in pregnant women and requires aggressive management and careful follow-up. Uncontrolled studies of the use of metronidazole in pregnancy indicate no increase in fetal loss or congenital abnormalities (17, 18).

Paramomycin is the luminal amebicide of choice in pregnant women, as it is a non-absorbable aminoglycoside. If there is no evidence of amebic liver abscess, therapy with erythromycin and paramomycin could be attempted, as erythromycin has a high level of success when used exclusively for amebic colitis. Follow-up stool examinations are essential to ensure eradication of the parasite.

Conclusion

Given the level of foreign travel and immigration from endemic areas, it is necessary for all physicians worldwide to be up-to-date regarding management of tropical diseases, or have ready access to information and expert physicians. By identifying areas of controversy and potential pitfalls in management, I hope to help physicians provide the best possible care for patients with *Entamoeba* infection and help researchers successfully address the current limitations in clinical practice.

References

1. Sargeaunt PG, Williams JE and Greene JD (1978). *Trans. R. Soc. Trop. Med. Hyg.* **72**: 519–521.
2. Jackson TFHG (1988). *Inter. J. Parasit.* **28**: 181–186.
3. Abd-Alla MD, Jackson TFGH and Gatherim V, *et al.* (1993). *J. Clin. Microbiol.* **31**: 2845–2850.
4. Haque R, Kress K and Wood S, *et al.* (1996). *J. Infect. Dis.* **15**: 752–755.
5. Britten D, Wilson SM and McNerney R, *et al.* (1997). *J. Clin. Microbiol.* **35**: 11–1111.
6. Mirelman D, Nuchamowitz Y and Stolarsky T (1997). *J. Clin. Microbiol.* **35**: 2405–2407.
7. Jackson TFHG (1987). *S. Afr. Med. J.* **72**: 657–658.
8. Nanda R, Baveja U and Anand BS (1984). *Lancet.* **2**: 301–303.
9. Jackson TFHG, Gathiram V and Simjee AE (1985). *Lancet.* **1**: 716–719.
10. Ravdin JI, Jackson TF and Petri Jr WA, *et al.* (1990). *J. Infect. Dis.* **162**: 768–772.
11. Gathiram V, Jackson TFHG and Ravdin JI (1987). *S. Afr. Med. J.* **72**: 669–672.
12. Abramowicz M, Editor (1998). *The Medical Letter.* **40**: 1–12.
13. Qureshi H, Ali A, Baqai R and Ahmed W (1997). *J. Intl. Med. Res.* **25**: 167–170.
14. Courtney KO, Thompson PE and Hodgkinson R, *et al.* (1960). *Ann. Biochem. Exp. Med.* **20 (Suppl)**: 449–456.

15. Sullam PM, Slutkin G and Gottlieb AB, *et al.* (1986). *Sex. Transm. Dis.* **13**: 151–155.
16. Abd-Alla M, El-Hawey AM and Ravdin JI (1992). *Amer. J. Trop. Med. Hyg.* **47**: 800–804.
17. Abou-El-Magd I, Soong CG, El-Hawey A.M and Ravdin JI (1996). *J. Infect. Dis.* **174**: 157–162.
18. Abd-Alla M, Jackson TGFH and Ravdin JI (1998). *Amer. J. Trop. Med. Hyg.* **49(supplement)**: 1993; 392.
19. Katzenstein D, Rickerson V and Braude A (1982). *Medicine (Baltimore).* **61**: 237–246.
20. Krogstad DJ, Spencer HC and Healy GR, *et al.* (1978). *Ann. Intern. Med.* **88**: 89–97.
21. Healy GR (1988). (Churchill Livingstone, New York), 635–649.
22. Irusen EM, Jackson TFGH and Simjee AE (1992). *Clin. Infect. Dis.* **14**: 889–893.
23. Jelinek T, Peyerl G, Löscher T and Nothdurft HD (1996). *Eur. J. Clin. Micro. Infect Dis.* **15**: 752–755.
24. Adams EB and MacLeod IN (1977). *Medicine (Baltimore).* **56**: 325–534.
25. Ralls PW, Barnes PF and Johnson MB, *et al.* (1987). *Radiology.* **165**: 805–807.
26. Van Sonnenberg E, Mueller PR and Schiffman RR, *et al.* (1985). *Radiology.* **156**: 631–635.
27. Morgan I (1978). *Int. J. Gynacol. Obstet.* **15**: 501.
28. Robinson SC and Mirchandani G (1966). *Am. J. Obstet. Gynecol.* **93**: 502.

Chapter 9

Unresolved and Open Questions in Research

David Mirelman

The Besen-Brender Chair of Microbiology and Parasitology
Department of Biological Chemistry
The Weizmann Institute of Science
Rehovot 76100, Israel

> Prophecy is the most gratuitous form of error
> George Eliot

Introduction

The most important goals in amebiasis research are the understanding and control of the parasite's pathogenicity and virulence. Investigations on the origins of pathogenicity of Entamoeba have been going on ever since the parasite was first discovered and described over one hundred years ago. One of the intriguing observations investigators made in those times was that human infection with *E. histolytica* could manifest itself either as an invasive, life threatening disease or, as in the majority of cases, in a symptomless form. Sellards and Walker (1) reported in 1913 that a considerable proportion (25%) of the human volunteers which they had experimentally infected with cysts isolated from an asymptomatic carrier, developed invasive disease whereas the others did not. Brumpt in 1925 (2) proposed that the two distinct possible courses of human infection (active disease or symptomless carriers) were caused by two different, albeit morphologically indistinguishable species of amebae which he termed *E. disenterii* (pathogenic) and *E. dispar* (non pathogenic). Brumpt's hypothesis could not be rigorously tested until the successful axenization of *Entamoeba histolytica*, by Diamond in the sixties (3), opened the way for modern molecular research of this parasite. Since then, significant advances have been achieved in many laboratories and it has become clear that *E. dispar* and *E. histolytica* are two different types of organisms (4). Nevertheless, a number of important questions, especially with respect to the molecular basis of pathogenicity, still remain to be clarified. In this chapter I will try to review and discuss some of the open issues which investigators in this field are currently trying to resolve.

Pathogenicity in Amebiasis: Is it genetic or acquired

A review of recent research accomplishments in Amebiasis would be incomplete if the controversial reports on ameba conversion from the nonpathogenic *E. dispar* type to the pathogenic *E. histolytica* form would not be discussed.

Interest in the differentiation between the nonpathogenic *E. dispar* and pathogenic *E. histolytica* strains was aroused in the '80s following Sargeaunt's observations on the correlation between the clinical picture of infected individuals and the pattern of the isoenzyme electrophoretic migration (zymogram) of amebic isolates that were morphologically indistinguishable (5). Over twenty different zymodemes were reported, most of which were isolated from asymptomatic cases. These intriguing findings aroused a worldwide interest to learn more about amebic virulence mechanisms and to compare in more detail the molecular biology of the different nonpathogenic *E. dispar* and pathogenic *E. histolytica* forms. The biggest problem in studying *E. dispar* was, and still is, difficulties in *in vitro* cultivation. In contrast to the pathogenic *E. histolytica* strains, *E. dispar* would not grow in the absence of bacterial cells or form colonies in soft agar (6). Considerable efforts were devoted to axenize *E. dispar* and during one of our attempts to wean a culture from its associated bacterial flora with antibiotics, we realized, completely unexpectedly, that the surviving trophozoites had somehow switched their zymodeme and started displaying all the biochemical and molecular characteristics of pathogenic *E. histolytica* (7). A similar conversion was observed with another *E. dispar* isolate, cloned by and obtained from P.G. Sargeaunt (8). Additional conversions were later confirmed with other *E. dispar* strains and independently reported by at least four unrelated research groups (9–12). Changes in isoenzyme electrophoretic mobilities of protozoan cells as a consequence of different growth medium or elimination of bacterial associates from the cultures was not a new phenomena and has been reported for cultures of *Paramecium, Tetrahymena* and *Trypanosoma cruzi* (13–15). Changes in the zymodeme of some *E. dispar* and *E. histolytica* isolates have been reported but were suggested to be due to changes in the starch content of the growth medium or to some unexplained genetic exchanges (16, 17). The various reports on the switching of zymodeme from an *E.dispar* to an *E. histolytica* pattern encountered, however, considerable skepticism among numerous investigators. A number of reasons have been cited; foremost were the various failed attempts by a number of investigators to repeat the conversion in culture of an *E. dispar* to an *E. histolytica* zymodeme as well as the inability to explain in molecular terms the significant genomic differences that were identified in the two forms of ameba, before and after the conversion. The failure to establish a more reproducible procedure for the conversion from an *E. dispar* to an *E. histolytica* zymodeme is indeed an unresolved problem. *E. histolytica* and especially *E. dispar* are fastidious organisms to cultivate and, for example, even though a procedure for axenization and an axenic growth medium were described for *E. histolytica* almost 30 years ago (3, 6), this is not trivial and to this day, axenization has been achieved by only a handful of investigators and the overall number of known axenic strains of *E. histolytica* is around twenty. Furthermore, it appears that none of the reported axenizations was ever done with precloned isolates and it is known that certain *E. histolytica* strains have also failed to grow axenically. In our lab there were quite a number of cases where *E. dispar* cultures did not convert their zymodeme and were able to grow in culture only if a small supplement of lethally irradiated bacterial cells was periodically added. Recently two other groups have shown that cultures of two strains of *E. dispar* could be axenized . The trophozoites grew slowly in the absence of other microbial cells and their zymodeme did not convert to that of an *E. histolytica* strain (18, 19). Another cited skepticism is with regard to the *E. dispar* cultures used in the successful conversion experiments. It has been suggested that the cultures in the reported experiments were inadvertently contaminated with *E. histolytica* trophozoites, which then outgrew the *E. dispar* cells whose growth rate was impaired as a result of weaning the associated bacteria by the antibiotics (20). *E. histolytica* trophozoites usually multiply faster than *E. dispar* in xenic cultures and, in experiments in which cultures of *E. dispar* were mixed with trophozoites of *E. histolytica*, even at a 10,000:1 ratio, the culture displayed a pathogenic zymodeme after 10 days in culture. Notwithstanding, if the argument of contamination is correct, the contaminating *E. histolytica* trophozoites should have outgrown the *E. dispar* also in the control cultures which were not treated with the antibiotics to eliminate the associated bacterial flora. This was never observed. Furthermore, although theoretically anything could be possible, it is highly unlikely that all five different laboratories that independently and unrelatedly reported conversions with at least eight different *E. dispar* isolates, were in all cases due to contamination artifacts.

As earlier mentioned, the most convincing argument why *E. dispar* and *E histolytica* are nowadays regarded as two different genetic species is due to the significant sequence differences that have been identified in numerous genes of the two forms of organisms (21–30). For example, the two pairs of hexokinase isoenzymes, whose different electrophoretic band mobility in *E. dispar* and *E. histolytica* had become one of the cornerstones of the zymodeme differentiation between the two types of amebae (5), were recently cloned, characterized and the recombinant enzymes expressed in bacteria (31). The amino acid sequences of the two hexokinase isoenzymes from *E. dispar* and *E. histolytica* differ and the different isoelectric values of the recombinant proteins nicely matched those of the isoenzymes previously isolated and characterized from the two types of amebae (32).

In view of the extensive molecular evidence in favor of two genetically different organisms, it is not surprising that it is difficult to accept the concept of zymodeme switching or ameba conversion in cultures. Undoubtedly the easiest way out of this controversy is to dismiss all these observations as an experimental artifact and forget the whole issue. On the other hand, for the few investigators who have witnessed conversions in their laboratories, it still is an intellectual challenge to try and find a clue to this enigma. In this connection it should be remembered that in comparison to other lower eukaryotes, research on the molecular biology of *Entamoebae* is still in its infancy and our present understanding is still very limited. Basic information such as the ploidy of *E. histolytica* is still unknown, and suggestions that they may have very high ploidy (>14n) and perhaps more than one genome have been raised. One of the hypothesis is that some types and most likely not all of *E. dispar* trophozoites, may harbor silent gene copies of the type that are normally present in the *E. histolytica* species. The transcription of such silent genes may sometimes be activated, for example, as a response to stress such as that of starvation for bacteria. Some indication that amebae may possess extranuclear organelles which contain DNA has been recently reported (33). In addition, sequences of the 145bp repetitive elements of the rDNA circular molecules, that are characteristic for *E. histolytica*, have been detected by PCR in two *E. dispar* strains (34, 35). In *Tetrahymena* it has been shown that depending on growth conditions, cells may amplify either one of the two types of rDNA episomes which they harbor (36). Furthermore, recently the gene coding a lysine-rich antigen specifically present on surfaces of *E. dispar* trophozoites was also found in an *E. histolytica* strain (37). These preliminary findings suggest that copies of genes, characteristic for one type of amebae, may sometimes be present in the other type. One of the main questions is how could they get there and be transferred from one type of ameba to the other? (i) Can amebae exchange genetic material either by rare sexual conjugation (17, 38, 39), transducing viruses or fusion events (40)? (ii) Can trophozoites, or some of the occasionally seen multinucleated amebae, carry a silent copy of an alternative gene or genome? (iii) Is virulence a truly genetically stable property (41–43)? We still need to know what, if any, role do the different viruses that were detected years ago (44) and which appear to be quite elusive, play in the molecular biology of *E. dispar* and *E. histolytica* cells. Furthermore, it will be important to elucidate the molecular contribution of bacteria to the amebae (45). Given the present technology, answers to some of the questions may be obtained with the new procedures for stable transfection (46–48) which enable the introduction of genetic markers into trophozoites of both species, as well as from the novel *in situ* detection techniques for identifying unique gene sequences (33). The ultimate answer, however, will undoubtedly come after completion of the sequencing of the entire genomes of *E. histolytica* (49) and *E. dispar*, a feat that will certainly be accomplished in coming years. Until then, it might be prudent to postpone any final judgment on the controversial isoenzyme switching or conversion phenomena.

Virulence of *E. histolytica*: Is it responsible for symptomatic and asymptomatic infections?

The clinical symptoms that are usually reported for individuals with proven infections of *E. histolytica* range from acute invasive disease to asymptomatic carriers (50). The majority of reported cases (~90%) however, consist of persons with mild or ill-defined intestinal symptoms which are usually not well documented and in many cases are considered asymptomatic. One of the main questions which has not yet been resolved is whether this wide spectrum of clinical manifestations is due to different infecting strains of *E. histolytica* and/or *E. dispar*, or to variations in host conditions. Many investigators are convinced that symptomatic infections are a consequence of a combination of both: a certain host susceptibility and a virulent strain.

The micro environmental conditions of the human colon are known to vary between different individuals in a number of parameters which can affect the growth of the parasite. First is the composition of their intestinal bacterial flora, which is a critical nutrient for the trophozoites and a contributor of enzymatic activities such as catalase (51) and hydrolases (52). The bacterial flora, which varies from individual to individual, also contributes to the overall redox potential, gas composition and pH of the colon. Second, mucus and sIgA secretions which protect the intestinal mucosal cells are also known to vary among hosts (53–55). The general physiological condition of the host also appears to be important and states of malnutrition as well as pregnancy have been shown to increase the chances of invasive amebiasis.

With respect to the parasite, *in vitro* cultured trophozoites of well characterized *E. histolytica* and *E. dispar* strains have also been shown to significantly differ in their relative virulence, as determined by various criteria such as: (i) the ability to induce the formation of liver lesions in rodents (56–59); (ii) the cytopathic effect as determined by the rate of destruction of tissue cultured monolayers of mammalian cells (51, 60–63) (iii) the rate of hemolysis and phagocytosis of human red blood cells (64–67), and (iv) their ability to resist lysis by complement (68–71). Virulence of axenically cultured trophozoites as well as their ability to resist lysis by complement are known to gradually decrease upon long term *in vitro* cultivation. Certain nutrient components such as different stocks of bovine serum or trypticase batches have been shown to affect growth and virulence (72). Periodic inoculation and recovery of trophozoites from a rodent liver lesion usually helps restore and maintain virulence. Virulence was also reported to be increased by reassociating the axenically grown trophozoites with certain bacteria (51, 73) or supplementing the growth medium with cholesterol (74), suggesting that the axenic cultures have a deficiency in certain critical nutrient components or factors which slowly affect the trophozoite's virulence. Preliminary observations comparing the virulence of strain HM-1:IMSS cultured for long term (2 months) in TYI-S-33 medium (6) containing two different batches of bovine serum, one with 90 mg/dL total cholesterol and the other 180 mg/dL, have shown that virulence was gradually lost in the cultures grown with the low cholesterol and maintained in the other (S. Moody-Haupt, unpublished observations).

A number of well characterized *E. histolytica* strains such as HK-9 and NIH-200 are less virulent than strain HM-1:IMSS, and strain Rahman has been shown to be completely avirulent in all *in vitro* assays (59). Interestingly, strain Rahman adheres very well to mammalian cell tissue cultures, but the virulence of this strain could not be restored by addition of cholesterol or reassociation with bacteria and it also did not produce lesions in hamsters even with inoculation of 5 million trophozoites per liver. The reasons for strain Rahman's lack of virulence have not yet been established, it would appear this is a mutant that has lost its virulence. Some *E. dispar* strains may not be completely avirulent and in some cases may display virulent properties, including the formation of small liver lesions in hamsters (59).

At the molecular level, virulence has been proposed to be due to three main amebic components: (i) a family of galactose-specific lectins which are the main adhesins that mediate the attachment of the trophozoite to galactose or N-acetyl galactosamine-containing glycoconjugates present on surfaces of mammalian cells (75, 76). The amebic cytopathic effect is inhibited and phagocytosis of mammalian cells are significantly reduced in the presence of galactose or N-acetyl galactosamine, indicating that the adherence process is an important prerequisite but not sufficient for the destruction of cells; (ii) the small, 77 amino acid pore-forming protein, known as amebapore (77–81) which damages the membrane integrity of mammalian target cells, and (iii) a family of cysteine proteinases, six of which (EhCP1-EhCP6) have been identified and partially characterized in *E. histolytica* (82, 83). Sequence analysis of the amebic CP enzymes revealed that they share considerable sequence homology (40–70%). The specific role of each of these cysteine proteinases has not yet been established (29, 82, 84). EhCP-3 (or ACP1 according to the nomenclature of Reed *et al.* (84)) was initially suggested as the one involved in virulence as it was not detected in *E. dispar* strains (84). Subsequent analysis revealed that a gene very similar to EhCP1 (or ACP-3) was present and transcribed in *E. dispar* (85, 86). Recently, another member of the cysteine proteinase family EhCP-5, was reported to be missing in *E. dispar* (82). This enzyme was shown to be associated with the trophozoite membranes and it has been proposed that it is the main proteinase involved in trophozoite virulence. The overall levels of cysteine proteinase activity as well as its secretion by intact trophozoites has been shown to vary among different strains of *E. histolytica* (87). Lysates of strain HK-9 have significantly lower levels of total cysteine proteinase activity than those of strain HM-1:IMSS. On the other hand, cysteine proteinase activity of lysates of the avirulent strain Rahman, including the levels of EhCP-5 transcripts, were found to be similar to that of strain HM-1:IMSS (Ankri *et al.* unpublished results). Moreover, in contrast to the intact trophozoites of strain Rahman, which do not have any cytopathic activity, trophozoite lysates of this strain destroy monolayers of tissue cultured mammalian cells as well as other lysates of virulent strains (88). The only lytic activity which appears to remain intact in trophozoites of strain Rahman, in contrast to that observed for *E. dispar* trophozoites, is their ability to lyse red blood cells (89). Our information about the *E. histolytica* hemolysin is still very limited (90). It appears not to require a thiol group (91) as it is not inhibited by cysteine proteinase inhibitors such as E-64 or allicin (92).

The role of the cysteine proteinases in virulence is currently being studied in trophozoites stably transfected with constructs containing genes coding for different cysteine proteinase genes. Preliminary results with trophozoites of virulent strain HM-1:IMSS, transfected in our lab (92a) with a construct encoding EhCP-5 antisense mRNA, show that the transcription and activity of most of the cysteine proteinases was significantly (~90%) ablated indicating that the antisense mRNA prevented the expression of most of the CP genes. Interestingly, the transfected trophozoites were not deficient in their cytopathic activity, as determined by their ability to destroy mammalian cell monolayers. As previously observed in strain HM-1:IMSS (93), addition of the cysteine proteinase inhibitor E-64 causes only a partial inhibition (50%) of destruction of monolayers suggesting that the activity of cysteine proteinases is not the only cause for the cytopathic effect. The activity of the hemolysin in the transfectants remained intact and unaffected by the antisense ablation of the cysteine proteinases. This is probably due to the fact that the sequence of the hemolysin transcript is significantly different from that of the other cysteine proteinase genes. These preliminary observations suggest that the cytopathic effect is mutifactorial and that the hemolysin could be one of the important molecular contributors to virulence.

Another type of molecule on trophozoite surfaces which seems to be involved in amebic virulence is the lipophosphoglycan (LPG) (94–96). We have recently demonstrated a correlation between the abundance of LPG and the virulence of a particular strain. Virulent trophozoites of strain HM-1:IMSS have high amounts of two types of closely related LPG's, whereas strain Rahman as well as strains of *E. dispar* are deficient in the composition and content of their cell surface lipophosphoglycan, and have less than 10% of the LPG content present in virulent strains. Interestingly, the less virulent trophozoites of strain HM-1:IMSS, grown in cholesterol-poor serum also demonstrated a deficiency in LPG components (96a). The molecular mechanisms by which LPG contributes to parasite virulence and how its synthesis and appearance on trophozoite surfaces is regulated are not yet known. An interesting possibility is that there may be a connection between the composition and structure of the LPG in the outer trophozoite surface and the presence of the putative, toxic molecules such as hemolysins, amebapore and CP's that appear to participate in the cytopathic effect. In trophozoites deficient in LPG, the assembly or exposure of toxic molecules may be impaired and fail to efficiently interact with target cells. A similar observation was recently reported for bacteria which lack lipopolysacharides (LPS) (97).

In summary, it appears that amebic virulence is the result of various molecular components, all of which are apparently needed for maximal effect. The elucidation of each of these virulence factors and the molecular mechanisms by which they interact with host cells and tissues is, and will continue to be, one of the most fascinating questions in amebic research.

Infections of *E. dispar* and *E. histolytica* in the same host

Numerous epidemiological studies, carried out mainly by Peter Sargeaunt's group (5, 38, 41, 98) using isoenzyme electrophoresis techniques (zymodeme) to differentiate between *E. dispar* and *E. histolytica* as well as more recent studies by others (99–102) using antibody based kits, have indicated that: (i) no *E. dispar* was ever found in an invasive case of symptomatic amebiasis, and (ii) individuals were never found to be infected simultaneously with both *E. histolytica* and *E. dispar*. Since these studies showed that a person could be infected with one but not both types of amebae, they reasoned that if *E. dispar* was found, the avirulent ameba would behave as a commensal and the infection would remain asymptomatic. In such situations there would be no need to treat the patient as he would never develop disease (41). This assertion had a lot of relevance for health authorities, especially for developing countries, as it could mean a very significant financial relief for their poorly funded health services. A number of investigators, however, were not convinced by this rather simplistic hypothesis, especially in view of the fact that it was quite well known that many individuals infected with *E. histolytica* harbored at the same time other nonpathogenic amebae such as *Entamoeba coli* or *Entamoeba moshkovsky*. It thus seemed odd that the morphologically indistinguishable *E. dispar* and *E. histolytica* would be mutually exclusive in the human host. In addition, quite a number of cases were reported where the infected individuals had high titers of antiamebic antibodies in their serum, possibly due to prior

E. histolytica infection, yet they were found to harbour only *E. dispar* trophozoites (103, 104). The recent introduction of very sensitive and accurate diagnostic tools in the form of PCR primers that are specific for *E. dispar* or *E. histolytica* (22, 27, 35, 105) has enabled the direct detection and characterization of the infecting parasite in the patient's stool, obviating the need for *in vitro* culture of the parasite for zymodeme determination (5). PCR techniques can detect one trophozoite of *E. histolytica* in the presence of a thousand fold of *E. dispar* and vice versa (106). In contrast, both zymodeme (5) and the existing ELISA based kits[100-102] were incapable of detecting the presence of small amounts (<100 trophs.) of *E. histolytica*. Using the newer PCR techniques, four different studies have recently shown that there is a high proportion of infected persons (20–70%, depending on the study) that harbor the two types of parasites at the same time (105, 107, 108). In a recent study of 48 asymptomatic Mexican schoolchildren, over 70% were found to have occult infections with *E. histolytica* (109). These preliminary findings raise a number of interesting and important questions and have lead to a reconsideration of earlier recommendations. First, it shows that only by PCR is it possible to detect mixed infections with *E. dispar* and *E. histolytica* and that ELISA methods may not be sufficiently sensitive. Second, zymodeme analyses, which requires a few days of *in vitro* cultivation of the ameba obtained from the stool before the electrophoretic analysis, are no longer to be used for differentiation because of poor sensitivity and possible culture selection of one or the other type of parasite. Current recommendations recently approved by the WHO (110, 111) state that whenever stools are found negative for *E. histolytica* , based on zymodeme or ELISA analysis, this should not be taken as sufficient proof that *E. histolytica* is not present or to determine that the patient should not be treated.

The presence of both types of parasites in the same patient could be one of the reasons for the variation in the degree of symptoms or for the sudden flare ups that many asymtomatic patients sometimes experience. It would be interesting to find out if this symptomological variation phenomenum is related to increases in the relative numbers of the virulent type of parasite present in the bowel of such patients. One of the problems in trying to answer such questions are the experimental limitations of studying the parasite's biology and behavior in the host. Experimental duplication of the ever-changing conditions that prevail in the human intestine is impossible and animal models are quite unreliable (54, 112, 113). Nevertheless, experiments designed to study the outcome of co-cultivation of both types of amebae under different conditions are currently under way. They are intended, among other things, to find out if *E. dispar* may have some effect on *E. histolytica* virulence and to establish whether genetic exchange exists between them, either by a rare sexual conjugation or fusion event.

Mysteries of the ameba genome

One of the most intriguing aspects of *E. histolytica* biology is the organization of its DNA. Significant variations have been observed in the DNA content and organization of the same strain under different growth conditions (114, 115). Chromosome-like structures have been observed by transmission electron microscopy, and molecular karyotypes have been obtained using pulsed field gel electrophoresis (25, 116, 117). Using these methodologies, large DNA molecules with different topology and electrophoretic properties have been identified (118–120). Coiled, relaxed and catenated circular as well as linear DNA molecules have been observed in *E. histolytica* (119, 121, 122). The existence of typical linear chromosomes has not yet been unequivocally confirmed and neither telomers nor centromers have been cloned (122). The first circular DNA molecules characterized have been the 25 Kb palindromic ribosomal DNA episomes which are present in more than 200 copies per trophozoite (123-125). rDNA gene copies have also been identified in linear DNA molecules (33). The high copy number of the rDNA genes and the presence of extranuclear DNA could be explained by an active self replication or amplification process. DNA regions within the circular rDNA molecules, which are able to replace the well established autonomous replication sequences (ARS) in yeast plasmids, have been identified (126, 127). An interesting recent observation by Orozco (128) suggests that the amplification of the rDNA circular molecules follows the onion skin model, whereby loops are formed by recombination of two non contiguous DNA strands. Bubble like forms, which undergo several rounds of replication, are generated from the recombinogenic region or from a putative replication origin. Circles or linear fragments are detached from the main DNA strand and these may recombine back with chromosome-like structures.

As was shown for other protozoans, the genome of *E. histolytica* appears to have considerable plasticity. Genomic polymorphisms and phenotypic variability have been reported (33, 129) but the molecular mechanisms of what appears to be non reciprocal recombination events, have yet to established. After relentless efforts, techniques for stable episomal transfection have been established in *Entamoeba* (46–48). On the other hand, homologous recombination and integration of exogenous DNA into the chromosome (for example in knockout experiments) has not yet been achieved. The reasons for this are most likely of a technical nature, but they again illustrate the unusual genome organization of this parasite.

Considerable progress has been achieved in recent years in the understanding of the regulation of gene transcription in *Entamoeba* (see Chapter V on Molecular Biology by Petri). What is not yet clear is whether novel molecular mechanisms such as RNA editing, which have been found in a number of protozoan parasites (130) may exist also in *Entamoeba*. Many of the genes in *E. histolytica* have been shown to be multicopy and small sequence differences were found in the coding regions of most of them (28, 131–135). Only three genes out of the more than thirty that have been characterized were reported to have introns (69, 136, 137). In addition, *Entamoeba* seem to have an as yet unclear mechanism for regulating gene expression at the translation level, and they are able to differentially express certain gene copies. Recent findings have shown that although the two gene copies, gLE3 and g34, of the ribosomal protein L-21 (RP-L21) are transcribed at equal levels, only one of them is actively translated (138–140). Moreover, an interesting difference was found: in *E. histolytica* the gene copy that is translated is gLE3 whereas in *E. dispar* it is g34 (138–140). The coding regions of the two RPL21 genes are almost identical, but significant sequence divergence (>50%) was found in the 5' and 3' untranslated regions of both genes, and investigations are under way to identify the different putative RNA binding factors in the UTR regions of the *E. histolytica* and *E. dispar* gene copies that may be responsible for the regulating mechanism.

In conclusion, the available information to date on the genome organization and regulation of gene expression in *Entamoeba* is still very limited. Preliminary observations indicate that it is quite unusual and very complex, considerable more work will be needed in order to unravel it.

Acknowledgments

Work from the author's laboratory was supported by grants from the Center for Molecular Biology of Tropical Diseases, and the Leo and Julia Forchheimer Center for Molecular Genetics, both at the Weizmann Institute of Science.

References

1. Sellards AW and Walker EL (1913). *The Philippine J. of Sci.* **VIII(4)**: 253.
2. Brumpt E (1925). *Bulletin de l'Académie Médicine (Paris)* **94**: 942.
3. Diamond LS (1968). *J. Parasitol.* **54**: 1047.
4. Diamond LS and Clark CG (1993). *J. Euk. Microbiol.* **40**: 340.
5. Sargeaunt PG *et al.* (1978). *Trans. R. Soc. Trop. Med. Hyg.* **72**: 519.
6. Diamond LS (1983). *Lumen dwelling protozoa: Entamoeba, Trichomonads and Giardia,* ed. Jensen JB (CRC Press, Boca Raton, FL) 65–109.
7. Mirelman D *et al.* (1986). *Exp. Parasitol.* **62**: 142.
8. Mirelman D *et al.* (1986). *Infect. Immun.* **65**: 827.
9. Mukherjee RM *et al.* (1993). *Trans. R. Soc. Trop. Med. Hyg.* **87**: 490.
10. Andrews BJ *et al.* (1990). *Trans. R. Soc. Trop. Med. Hyg.* **84**: 63.
11. Vargas MA and Orozco E (1993). *Parasitol. Res.* **79**: 353.
12. Vrchotova N *et al.* (1993). *Ann. Parasitol. Hum. Comp.* **68**: 67.
13. Allen SL (1968). *Ann. N.Y. Acad. Sci.* **151**: 190.
14. Rowe E *et al.* (1970). *Biochem. Genetics* **5**: 151.
15. Alves AMB *et al.* (1993). *Exp. Parasitol.* **77**: 246.
16. Blanc D and Sargeaunt PG (1991). *Exp. Parasitol.* **72**: 87.
17. Blanc D. *et al.* (1989) *Trans. R. Soc. Trop. Med. Hyg.* **83**: 787.
18. Takeuchi T and Kobayashi S (1997). *Arch. Med. Res. (Mexico)* **28**: 108.
19. Clark CG (1995). *J. Euk. Microbiol.* **42**: 590.
20. Clark CG and Diamond LS (1993). *Exp. Parasitol.* **77**: 456.
21. Edman U *et al.* (1990). *J. Exp. Med.* **172**: 879.
22. Clark CG and Diamond LS (1991). *Mol. Biochem. Parasitol.* **49**: 297.
23. Garfinkel LI *et al.* (1989). *Infect. Immun.* **57**: 926.
24. McKerrow JH *et al.* (1993). *Ann. Rev. Microbiol.* **47**: 821.
25. Petter R *et al.* (1993). *Infect. Immun.* **61**: 3574.
26. Stanley SLJ *et al.* (1990). *Proc. Natl. Acad. Sci. USA* **87**: 4976.
27. Tannich E *et al.* (1991). *Mol. Biochem. Parasitol.* **49**: 61.
28. Tannich E *et al.* (1989). *Proc. Natl. Acad. Sci. USA* **86**: 5118.
29. Tannich E *et al.* (1991). *J. Biol. Chem.* **266**: 4798.
30. Torian BE *et al.* (1990). *Proc. Natl. Acad. Sci. USA* **87**: 6358.
31. Ortner (1997). *Mol. Biochem. Parasitol.* **86**: 85.
32. De Meester F *et al.* (1990). *Infect. Immun.* **58**: 1396.
33. Orozco E (1997). *Mol. Gen. Genet.* **254**: 250.
34. Orozco E (1992). *Infect. Agents and Dis.* **1**: 19.
35. Mirelman D *et al.* (1990). *Infect. Immun.* **58**: 1660.
36. Bruns PJ *et al.* (1985). *Proc. Natl. Acad. Sci. USA* **82**: 2844.

37. Bracha R *et al.* (1995). *Infect. Immun.* **63**: 917.
38. Sargeaunt PG (1985). *Trans. Roy. Soc. Trop. Med. Hyg.* **79**: 86.
39. Sargeaunt PG *et al.* (1988). *Trans. R. Soc. Trop. Med. Hyg.* **82**: 862.
40. Solis F and Orozco E (1991). *Exp. Parasitol.* **72**: 236.
41. Allason-Jones E *et al.* (1986). *N. Engl. J. Med.* **315**: 353.
42. Mirelman D *et al.* (1984). *Exp. Parasitol.* **57**: 172.
43. Goldmeier D *et al.* (1986). *Lancet* **1**: 641.
44. Diamond LS *et al.* (1972). *J. Virol.* **9**: 326.
45. Rosenthal B (1997). *J. Bacteriol.* **179**: 3736.
46. Vines RR *et al.* (1995). *Mol. Biochem. Parasitol.* **71**: 265.
47. Nickel R and Tannich E (1994). *Proc. Natl. Acad. Sci. USA* **91**: 7095.
48. Moshitch-Moshkovitch S *et al.* (1997). *Mol. Biochem. Parasitol.* **83**: 257.
49. Azam A *et al.* (1996). *Gene* **28**: 113.
50. Walsh JA (1988). *Amebiasis: Human Infection by Entamoeba histolytica*, ed. Ravdin JI (Wiley Medical, N.Y.).
51. Bracha R and Mirelman D (1984). *J. Exp. Med.* **160**: 353.
52. Variyam EP (1992). *Arch. Med. Res (Mexico)* **23**: 223.
53. Tse SK and Chadee K (1992). *Infect. Immun.* **60**: 1603.
54. Leitch GJ *et al.* (1988). *Am. J. Trop. Med. Hyg.* **39**: 282.
55. Belley A *et al.* (1996). *Gastroenterology* **111**: 1484.
56. Espinosa Cantellano M *et al.* (1997). *Arch. Med. Res. (Mexico)* **28**: 204.
57. Chadee K and Meerovitch E (1984). *Am. J. Pathol.* **117**: 71.
58. Tsutsumi V *et al.* (1984). *Am. J. Pathol.* **117**: 81.
59. Burchard GD and Mirelman D (1988). *Exp. Parasitol.* **66**: 231.
60. Ravdin JI and Guerrant RL (1981). *J. Clin. Invest.* **68**: 1305.
61. Mirelman D and Kobiler D (1981). *Adhesion properties of Entamoeba histolytica* (Ciba Symp., Pitman Medical, Tunbridge Wells, England) 1–17.
62. Munguia BC *et al.* (1997). *Arch. Med. Res. (Mexico)* **28**: 116.
63. Martinez-Palomo A *et al.* (1985). *J. Protozool.* **32**: 166.
64. Trissl D *et al.* (1978). *Arch. Invest. Med (Mexico)* **9**: 219.
65. Bailey GB *et al.* (1987). *Infect. Immun.* **55**: 1848.
66. Mukherjee RM *et al.* (1991). *J. Diarrhoeal Dis. Res.* **9**: 11.
67. Montfort I and Perez-Tamayo R (1994). *Parasitol. Today* **7**: 271.
68. Reed SL *et al.* (1983). *Trans. R. Soc. Trop. Med. Hyg.* **77**: 248.
69. Urban B *et al.* (1996). *Mol. Biochem. Parasitol.* **80**: 171.
70. Hamelmann C *et al.* (1993). *Parasite Immunol.* **15**: 223.
71. Hamelmann C *et al.* (1993). *Infect. Immun.* **61**: 1636.
72. Diamond LS (1993). *J. Protozool* **38**: 211.

73. Bracha R and Mirelman D (1983). *Infect. Immun.* **40**: 882.
74. Lujan HD and Diamond LS (1997). *Arch. Med. Res (Mexico)* **28**: 96.
75. Petri WAJ and Schnaar RL (1995). *Methods Enzymol.* **253**: 98.
76. Ravdin JI *et al.* (1988). *Amebiasis: Human Infection by Entamoeba histolytic,* ed. Ravdin JI (John Wiley & Sons, N.Y.).
77. Lynch EC *et al.* (1982). *Embo J.* **1**: 801.
78. Gitler C and Mirelman D (1986). *Ann. Rev. Microbiol.* **40**: 237.
79. Leippe M *et al.* (1994). *Mol. Microbiol.* **14**: 895.
80. Leippe M *et al.* (1994). *Proc. Natl. Acad. Sci. USA* **91**: 2602.
81. Andrä J *et al.* (1997). *Arch. Med. Res. (Mexico)* **28**: 156.
82. Bruchhaus I *et al.* (1996). *Mol. Microbiol.* **22**: 255.
83. Reed SL *et al.* (1993). *J. Clin. Invest.* **91**: 1532.
84. Reed SL (1989). *J. Clin. Microbiol.* **27**: 2772.
85. Bruchhaus I and Tannich E (1996). *Parasitol. Res.* **82**: 189.
86. Mirelman D *et al.* (1996). *Mol. Biochem. Parasitol.* **78**: 47.
87. Keene WE *et al.* (1990). *Exp. Parasitol.* **71**: 199.
88. Lopez-Revilla R (1980). *Am. J. Trop. Med. Hyg.* **29**: 209.
89. Trissl D (1978). *J. Exp. Med.* **148**: 1137.
90. Keller F (1988). *J. Protozool.* **35**: 359.
91. Rosales-Encina JL *et al.* (1992). *Arch. Med. Res. (Mexico)* **23**: 243.
92. Ankri S *et al.* (1997). *Antimicrob. Agents Chem.* **41**: 2286.
    (a) Ankri S *et al.* (1998). *Mol. Microbiol.* **28**: 777–785.
93. Li E *et al.* (1994). *Infect. Immun.* **62**: 5112.
94. Moody S *et al.* (1997). *Parasitology* **114**: 95.
95. Bhattacharya A *et al.* (1992). *Mol. Biochem. Parasitol.* **56**: 161.
96. Stanley, Jr. SL *et al.* (1992). *Mol. Biochem. Parasitol.* **50**: 127.
    (a) Moody S *et al.* (1998) *J. Euk Microbiol.* **45**: 179–182.
97. Rahman MM *et al.* (1997). *J. Bacteriol.* **179**: 2126.
98. Sargeaunt PG (1987). *Parasitol. Today* **3**: 40.
99. Ravdin JI (1994). *Gut* **35**: 1018.
100. Haque R *et al.* (1993). *J. Infect. Dis.* **167**: 247.
101. Haque R *et al.* (1994). *Am. J. Trop. Med. Hyg.* **50**: 595.
102. Haque R *et al.* (1995). *J. Clin. Microbiol.* **33**: 2558.
103. Jackson TFHG *et al.* (1985). *Lancet* **i**: 716.
104. Jetter A *et al.* (1997). *Arch. Med. Res. (Mexico)* **28**: 319.
105. Walderich B *et al.* (1995) European Conference on Tropical Medicine (Blackwell Science, Hamburg) Abs. L119.
106. Mirelman D *et al.* (1997). *J. Clin. Microbiol.* **35**: 2405.
107. Romero JL *et al.* (1992). *Arch. Med. Res. (Mexico)* **23**: 277.

108. Acuna-Soto R *et al.* (1993). *Am. J. Trop. Med. Hyg.* **48**: 58.
109. Newton-Sanchez OA *et al.* (1997). *Arch. Med. Res.* **28**: 311.
110. World Health Organization (1997). *Epidemiological Bulletin*, in PAHO, Geneva, pp. 13–14.
111. World Health Organization (1997). *Amoebiasis*, in Weekly Epidemiological Record, Geneva, pp. 97–100.
112. Leitch GJ *et al.* (1985). *Infect. Immun.* **47**: 68.
113. Leitch GJ (1988). *Am. J. Trop. Med. Hyg.* **38**: 480.
114. Sharma NN *et al.* (1969). *J. Protozool.* **16**: 405.
115. Lopez-Revilla R and Gómez R (1978). *Exp. Parasitol.* **44**: 243.
116. Orozco E *et al.* (1993). *Mol. Biochem. Parasitol.* **59**: 29.
117. Baez-Camargo M *et al.* (1997). *Arch. Med. Res. (Mexico)* **28**: 8.
118. Dhar SK *et al.* (1995). *Mol. Biochem. Parasitol.* **70**: 203.
119. Lioutas C *et al.* (1995). *Exp. Parasitol.* **80**: 349.
120. Báez-Camargo M *et al.* (1996). *Mol. Gen. Genet.* **253**: 289.
121. Baez-Camargo M *et al.* (1997). *Anal. Lett.* **29**: 745.
122. Flores E *et al.* (1997). *Arch. Med. Res. (Mexico)* **28**: 5.
123. Huber M *et al.* (1989). *Mol. Biochem. Parasitol.* **32**: 285.
124. Cazares F *et al.* (1994). *Mol. Microbiol.* **12**: 607.
125. Bhattacharya S *et al.* (1989). *J. Protozool.* **36**: 365.
126. Lohia A *et al.* (1990). *Gene* **96**: 197.
127. Grodberg J *et al.* (1990). *Nucl. Acids Res.* **18**: 5515.
128. Orozco E *et al.* (1997). *Arch. Med. Res. (Mexico)* **28**: 24.
129. de M. Feitosa L *et al.* (1997). *Arch. Med. Res.(Mexico)* **28**: 27.
130. Stuart K (1997). *Microbiol. Mol. Biol. Rev.* **61**: 105.
131. Ramakrishnan G *et al.* (1996). *Mol. Microbiol.* **19**: 91.
132. Ortner S *et al.* (1995). *Mol. Biochem. Parasitol.* **73**: 189.
133. Mann BJ *et al.* (1991). *Proc. Natl. Acad. Sci. USA* **88**: 3248.
134. McCoy JB *et al.* (1993). *Mol. Biochem. Parasitol.* **61**: 325.
135. Purdy JE *et al.* (1993). *Mol. Biochem. Parasitol.* **62**: 53.
136. Plaimauer B (1994). *Mol. Biochem. Parasitol.* **66**: 181.
137. Lohia A and Samuelson J (1993). *Gene* **127**: 203.
138. Petter R *et al.* (1992). *Mol. Biochem. Parasitol.* **56**: 329.
139. Petter R *et al.* (1994). *Gene* **150**: 181.
140. Moshitch-Moshkovitch S *et al.* (1998). *Mol. Microbiol.* **27**: 677.

University of California